Mathematical Methods in Immunology

Courant Lecture Notes in Mathematics

Executive Editor
Jalal Shatah

Managing Editor
Copy Editor
Paul D. Monsour

Production Editor
Reeva Goldsmith

Jerome K. Percus

Courant Institute of Mathematical Sciences

23 Mathematical Methods in Immunology

Courant Institute of Mathematical Sciences
New York University
New York, New York

American Mathematical Society
Providence, Rhode Island

2010 *Mathematics Subject Classification.* Primary 92–XX.

———————————————————————

For additional information and updates on this book, visit
www.ams.org/bookpages/cln-23

———————————————————————

Library of Congress Cataloging-in-Publication Data

Percus, Jerome K. (Jerome Kenneth)
   Mathematical methods in immunology / Jerome K. Percus.
      p. cm. — (Courant lecture notes in mathematics ; v. 23)
   Includes bibliographical references and index.
   ISBN 978-0-8218-7556-8 (alk. paper)
   I. American Mathematical Society.   II. Title.   III. Series: Courant lecture notes in mathematics ; 23. 1529-9031 [DNLM: 1. Immunologic Techniques.   2. HIV—immunology.   3. Immunity, Innate.   4. Models, Theoretical.   QW525]

616.97′92079—dc23

2011045038

———————————————————————

Contents

Preface

Back in the mid-1980s, I felt that immunology was an increasingly important field that might profit from appropriate mathematical analysis and made the obvious move: I developed and taught a course on the topic. It soon became clear that most of what I regarded as the valuable insights were due to one person: Alan Perelson, at Los Alamos, and so I contacted Alan, initiating a period of occasional collaboration that kept me informed of what had been discovered and what was being done about it. One result was that when I repeated this course every few years, it had the benefit of considerable new material. The last extensive rewriting was in 2002, and this, with embarrassingly few updates, represents the material presented in these lecture notes.

The topic coverage in a one-semester course on quantitative aspects of a large field must involve compromises and have a restricted scope. Here, this was accomplished by focusing in the main on the battle between the HIV virus and the adaptive immune system. This means that, on the biology side, the rapidly expanding study of the innate immune system and the role of inflammatory response are simply ignored, a dangerous but necessary tactic. The topics of allergy and autoimmunity—among others—are absent as well. And of course, the roles of organisms normally associated—largely internally—with that of the mammalian systems that are implicitly our focus, are not even mentioned. On the more mathematical side, much of the material presented is in the "classical" format of population dynamics of a well-mixed population—translating at once to chemical kinetics. However, the balance is partially redressed by a number of excursions into small and/or discrete populations, making initial contact with the ubiquity of fluctuations, driving much of current research.

It goes without saying that advantage was taken of the talents of a number of individuals—many of Alan Perelson's collaborators, as well as Ora Percus, who is responsible for a good deal of the content and for the elimination of numerous ambiguities and non-sequiturs. And Daisy Mojar-Calderon, who converted my illegible scrawlings into material of potential value.

CHAPTER 1

The HIV Pandemic

1.1. Introduction

When our immune system is compromised, it is only a matter of time before the numerous pathogens that surround us wreak their deadly damage. One of the most effective adversaries that the immune system may have to face is the HIV class of viruses, which targets some of its principal components. We will not go into great detail as to the precise fashion in which it does so, in part because this knowledge remains quite incomplete. We will focus instead on more general characteristics of the time development of the interacting virus and cell populations as an example of the thought processes that are useful in putting such biological events into a quantitative framework. In this chapter, we will also introduce a number of incompletely defined biological terms, reserving details for the thoroughly descriptive Chapter 2.

A virus is composed of a relative short string of genes (or perhaps two strings in parallel), normally protected by protein, and in the case of HIV surrounded by a lipid membrane. It infects a cell by binding to it via receptor molecules on the cell surface, and then injects its genes into the cell; they infiltrate the cell's manufacturing facility and cause it to produce more copies of the virus's genome (its string of genes) and proteins, which assemble and bud out of the cell as new viruses. A DNA virus simply inserts its DNA genome into the cell's DNA, while an RNA virus requires reverse transcriptase from the virus to construct its usable DNA. HIV, aside from its target, which is primarily a helper T-cell, a mainstay of the immune system, goes about its business pretty much like any other RNA virus, as cartooned in Figure 1.1. It binds to a cell via the cell's CD4 receptor, among others, injects its RNA through the cell membrane into the cell cytoplasm, the RNA produces a DNA copy which passes through the nuclear membrane, is integrated into the host DNA, and waits. When the T-cell is activated, which is bound to happen if it responds to an infection, all elements of the virus are manufactured, together with much of the cell's own needs; many of the viral proteins are made as one big string. This is then cleaved by proteases to produce the functional proteins of the virus, and the self-assembled virus (or "virion," used interchangeably to denote a single viral particle) leaves the cell by punching its way out.

Under drug-free conditions, HIV infection, once developed, is nonetheless held almost completely in check by the host immune system. This marvel of evolution, which we will later examine in great detail, both kills infected cells and digests viral particles. During the long (5- to 15-year) period of control, which gradually

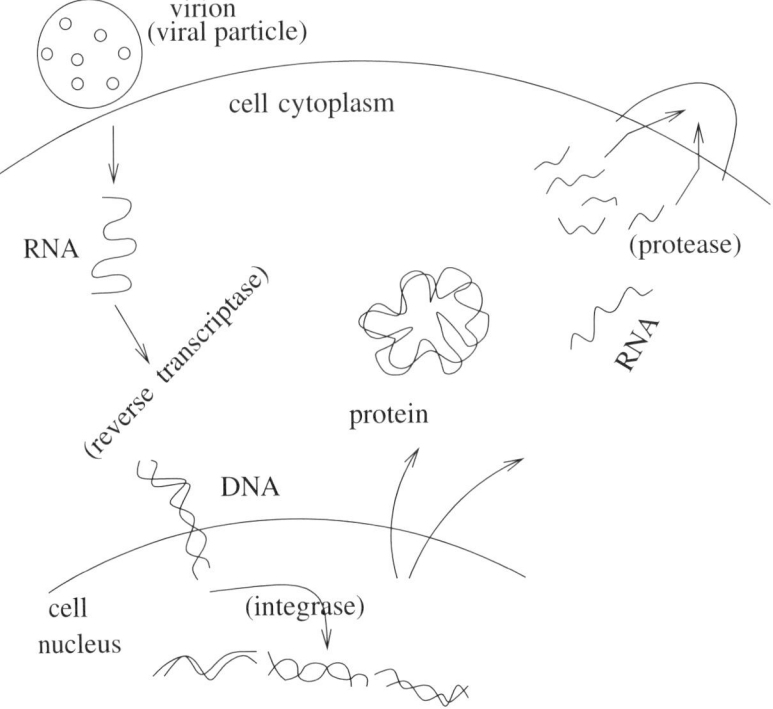

FIGURE 1.1. Major events in initial HIV infection.

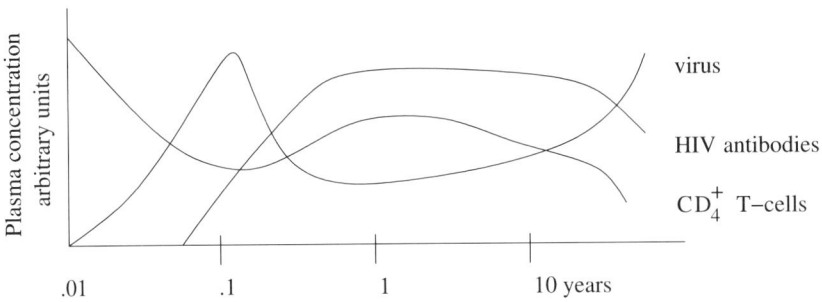

FIGURE 1.2. Typical time development of HIV infection.

weakens, the host is in an almost steady asymptomatic state, and it is during this period that one stands a better chance of understanding the population dynamics of the joint virus-immune system, hoping in this way to rationalize pharmaceutical treatment.

1.2. Prototype Dynamics

There are very rapid changes in viral and immune cell populations during the first few months of infection. We will attend mainly to the long, seemingly steady-state asymptomatic period that follows (Figure 1.2), the sustained levels normally referred to as the *set point*. A big hint as to what is going on in steady state stems

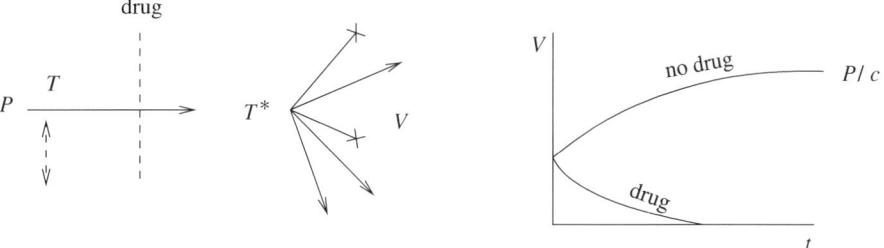

FIGURE 1.3. Effect of ideal drug treatment.

from the clinical observation that treatment with a powerful antiretroviral drug, thereby removing the source of new virus, results in rapid exponential decrease of virus. This strongly suggests that the virus population $V(t)$ is being controlled by a combination of constant source P (every T-cell gets zapped by virus, producing an infected T-cell T*, which spews forth virus), an effective clearance rate for virus:

$$\frac{dV}{dt} = P - cV.$$

A completely efficient drug (Figure 1.3) would make $P = 0$ so that $V(t) = V(0)e^{-ct}$, and clinical data results in $1/c = 1$ hour. Given this, then in steady state without the drug, $0 = P - cV$, and estimates of $V(0)$ allow us to estimate $P \sim 10^{10}$ virions/day. Since drug efficiency is less than 100%, we have an overestimate for $1/c$ (c really has to be higher than observed, to take care of the remnant of P).

The above argument leaves unexplained both the contributions to the viral growth rate and the size of the T-cell population that unwittingly serves as the source of virus. For these, we need a more detailed model. Let us refer all populations to some unit volume (generally taken in the business as $1 \ \mu\ell = 1 \ mm^3$). Then, to start, we distinguish between the susceptible but uninfected T-cell population $T(t)$, and the population $T^*(t)$ that has been successfully ("productively") infected. The uninfected T's will be modeled via a source s, a natural death rate d, and a rate at which they become infected, taken (as in the chemical kinetics law of mass action) as proportional both to the viral concentration and T-cell concentration:

(1.1a)
$$\frac{dT}{dt} = s - dT - kVT.$$

The infected T's are of course produced at the same rate kVT, and have their own natural death rate δ after infection:

(1.1b)
$$\frac{dT^*}{d\tau} = kVT - \delta T^*.$$

The infected cells are indeed the source of new virions, but each T^* can churn out a large number, say $N \sim 10^2 - 10^4$, of virions before dying, so now

(1.1c)
$$\frac{dV}{dt} = N\delta T^* - cV.$$

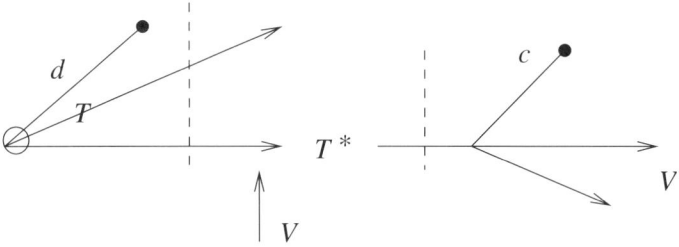

FIGURE 1.4. Schematic representation of interacting populations.

Schematically, one can represent the situation as in Figure 1.4 with drug interference locations shown dotted, and more succinctly in the notation of chemical
reactions:

$$O \xrightarrow{s} T, \quad T \xrightarrow{d} \bullet,$$

$$T + V \xrightarrow{k} T^*$$

$$T^* \xrightarrow{\delta} NV, \quad V \xrightarrow{c} \bullet.$$

This basic model of three coupled ODEs is fairly simple but not analytically
trivial, and it is worth looking at some extreme cases to get a feeling for its properties. To do so, we must decide what "extreme" means; after all, there are six
parameters to play with. Since there are three concentration variables and one time
variable, we can choose units so that two of the rate contributions in each equation have the same coefficient, and one of the time derivatives as well. Scaling as
$T = \alpha\tau, T^* = \alpha^*\tau^*, V = \beta v$, and $t = \gamma t'$, we have

$$\frac{\alpha}{\gamma}\frac{d\tau}{dt'} = s - d\alpha\tau - k\beta\alpha v\tau,$$

$$\frac{\alpha^*}{\gamma}\frac{d\tau^*}{dt'} = h\beta\alpha v\tau - \alpha^*\delta\tau^*,$$

$$\frac{\beta}{\gamma}\frac{dv}{dt'} = n\delta\alpha^*\tau^* - c\beta v,$$

and so choosing $d\alpha = k\beta\alpha$, $k\beta\alpha = \alpha^*\delta$, and $\beta/\gamma = N\delta\alpha^* = c\beta$, or

$$\beta = \frac{d}{k}, \quad \gamma = \frac{1}{c}, \quad \alpha^* = \frac{cd}{N\delta k}, \quad \alpha = \frac{c}{Nk},$$

there results the canonical form

(1.2a)
$$\frac{c}{d}\frac{d\tau}{dt'} = a - \tau - v\tau,$$

(1.2b)
$$\frac{c}{\delta}\frac{d\tau^*}{dt'} = v\tau - \tau^*,$$

(1.2c)
$$\frac{dv}{dt'} = \tau^* - v,$$

where $a = \frac{Nk}{cd}s$. Note that time has now been scaled by that of the viral dynamics.

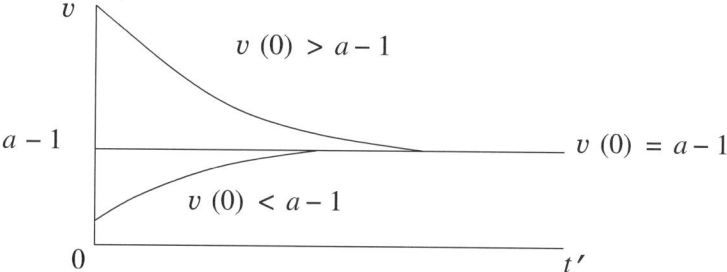

FIGURE 1.5. Time course for condition (1) when $a > 1$.

Actually, clinical estimates give

$$c \sim 23/\text{day}, \quad d \sim .01/\text{day}, \quad \delta \sim 1/\text{day}$$

but let us ignore these "details" in our enumeration of extremes. A first extreme might be the assumption that $c/\delta \to \infty$; then (1.2b) implies $\tau^* = \text{const}$, reducing (1.2c) to the primitive case we previously examined.

The opposite and more questionable extreme is $c/\delta \to 0$. This says that reaction (1.2b) remains in "equilibrium," being fed by (1.2a) and feeding (1.2c); as the Michaelis-Menten condition for intermediates, it is often used and often valid. There are now two "subextremes":

(1) $c/d \to 0$ as well, in which case both τ and τ^* can be solved for in (1.2a) and (1.2b), and substituted into (1.2c),

$$(1.3) \qquad \frac{dv}{dt'} = v \frac{a - (1 + v)}{1 + v},$$

stationary at the values $v_0 = 0$ or $v_0 = a - 1$. Solution of this single ODE is routine (do it). If $a > 1$, it is best written as

$$|v - (a - 1)| = K v^{1/a} e^{-t'(a-1)/a},$$

and if a is really large (Figure 1.5), as

$$|v - (a - 1)| \sim K e^{-t'}.$$

Thus, high initial v settles exponentially to $a - 1$, typical perhaps of the approval to steady state that we have seen. On the other hand, if $a < 1$, we write instead

$$v = K'(v + 1 - a)^a e^{-(1-a)t'},$$

so that for really small a (remember: $a = Nks/cd$ is an overall production rate divided by an overall destruction rate)

$$v \sim K' e^{-t'},$$

the infection being quenched.

(2) The second subextreme is $c/d \to \infty$, in which case $\tau = \text{const}$, and one has instead

$$\frac{dv}{dt'} = (\tau - 1)v,$$

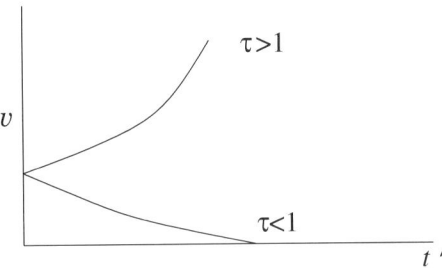

FIGURE 1.6. Time course for condition (2).

showing (Figure 1.6) for $\tau > 1$ an unstable divergence in v whenever the source τ is large enough and decay when $\tau < 1$. Here, viral production is controlled by the number of cells available to be infected.

Perhaps we should instead say nothing about $p = c/d$, in which case (1.2a) and (1.2b) become

$$(1.4) \qquad \begin{aligned} p\frac{d\tau}{dt'} &= a - \tau - v\tau, \\ \frac{dv}{dt'} &= (\tau - 1)v. \end{aligned}$$

Now, there is a nontrivial repertoire, and we have the opportunity of trotting out a little more standard mathematical machinery. The interesting case is that of $a > 1$, and we would like to know, for example, what the system settles down to at long time. Stationary solutions, i.e., $0 = a - \tau - v\tau$, $0 = (\tau - 1)v$, certainly exist:

$$\begin{cases} \tau_0 = 1 \\ v_0 = a - 1 \end{cases} \quad \text{or} \quad \begin{cases} \tau_0 = a \\ v_0 = 0 \end{cases}$$

but is either one stable? To find out, we perturb the stationary state, $\tau = \tau_0 + \Delta\tau$, $v = v_0 + \Delta v$, and write out the dynamics to first order in the perturbation:

$$\begin{aligned} p\frac{d\Delta\tau}{dt'} &= -(1 + v_0)\Delta\tau - \tau_0\Delta v, \\ \frac{d\Delta v}{dt'} &= v_0\Delta\tau + (\tau_0 - 1)\Delta v. \end{aligned}$$

As a pair of homogeneous linear equations, the elementary solutions have the form

$$\begin{pmatrix} \Delta\tau(t') \\ \Delta v(t') \end{pmatrix} = \begin{pmatrix} c_\tau \\ c_v \end{pmatrix} e^{\lambda t'}$$

for suitable constants c_τ, c_v, and λ, and we can write

$$\begin{pmatrix} p\lambda + 1 + v_0 & -\tau_0 \\ v_0 & \lambda + 1 - \tau_0 \end{pmatrix} \begin{pmatrix} c_\tau \\ c_v \end{pmatrix} = 0,$$

solvable if the coefficient determinant vanishes:

$$p\lambda^2 + \lambda(1 + v_0 - p(\tau_0 - 1)) + 1 + v_0 - \tau_0 = 0.$$

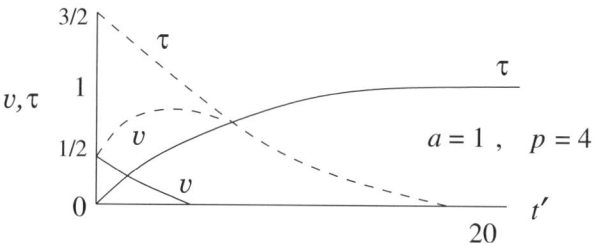

FIGURE 1.7. Time course when $c = 4d$, $a = 1$.

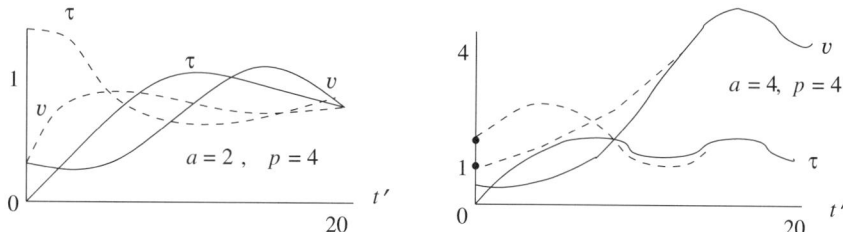

FIGURE 1.8. Cases $a = 2$ and $a = 4$.

The available values of λ for the above two stationary points are then

$$\lambda = \frac{1}{2p}\left(-a \pm \sqrt{a^2 - 4(a-1)p}\right), \quad \lambda = \left\{-\frac{1}{p}, a - 1\right\}.$$

Let us first polish off the weak source, $a < 1$, case. Since $v(t')$, satisfying $d \ln v(t')/dt' = \tau(t') - 1$ from (1.4), can never get negative (the integral over t' of $d \ln v(t')/dt'$ cannot get to $-\infty$), the first stationary point, with $v_0 = a - 1 < 0$, is not accessible. The second one is, and the two possible exponents λ in $e^{\lambda t'}$ are both negative. Thus, the virus is eliminated, $v_0 = 0$, at long time, and any perturbation dies out. The $a = 1$ case is marginal, and which stationary solution is achieved depends upon initial conditions. For example, for $v(0) = \frac{1}{2}$ and $\tau(0) = 0$ or $\tau(0) = \frac{3}{2}(\cdots)$ at $p = 4$, we have the results pictured in Figure 1.7. But for $a > 1$, the second stationary point yields a perturbation solution with one positive exponent, so that unless the perturbation is tuned impossibly carefully, it will necessarily diverge at first and set the dynamics on the path to the fully stable solution at the elevated virus concentration $a - 1$. Note that at $p > a/4$ (Figure 1.8), the path to the stable high virus state is expected to oscillate, since each λ is complex.

1.3. Effect of Drug Treatment

A leading problem is how to interfere with, or reverse, the progression of HIV infection to a high-V, low-T state. Of course, this is a matter of increasing the death rate of viable virus, decreasing its birth rate, or both. We will look first at external interference, and then at interference by other components of the immune system.

Let us now drop the Michaelis-Menten intermediate equilibrium approximation in favor of the tacit assumption that the T-cell population is invariant in time, which would indeed be the case for $c/d \to \infty$ in our model. In fact, one knows that this population is under tight homeostatic control, which is another way of saying that the source strength s depends upon the population level (as well, of course, as on the depletion rate—see later). Although there is certainly a time lag in the resetting of s, it is not unreasonable to imagine that the concentration $T(t)$ is fixed at some T_0 and later on drop this strict assumption. And this substantially simplifies the ensuing analysis: In unscaled form, our system is now represented by

(1.5)
$$\frac{dT^*}{dt} = -\delta T^* + k T_0 V,$$
$$\frac{dV}{dt} = N\delta T^* - cV,$$

a strictly linear pair of homogeneous ODEs with $T_0^* = 0$, $V_0 = 0$, as the only stationary state except for the very special setting $NkT_0 = c$. The question is whether this state is stable or unstable.

We'll scale a bit differently from our previous treatment: now take $\alpha = \alpha^* = 1$, $\beta = N\delta/c$, $\gamma = 1/c$, leading to

(1.6) $q\dot{\tau}^* = -\tau^* + bv, \quad \dot{v} = \tau^* - v,$

$$\text{where } q = \frac{c}{\delta}, \ b = \frac{NkT_0}{c}, \ a = \left(\frac{s}{dT_0}\right)b,$$

and d/dt' is denoted by an upper dot. Note that in the absence of virus, our previous T-dynamics would have given the stationary state $T_0 = s/d$, so that if this value were retained, b would reduce to the source strength a of the previous notation. At any rate, the dynamics of the above pair will be a linear combination of two exponentials whose exponents now satisfy (show this)

(1.7) $q\lambda^2 + (q+1)\lambda + 1 - b = 0.$

Without even solving, it is clear that there will be two negative λ's if $b < 1$, and the system will sink to $\tau^* = v = 0$; but one λ will be positive if $b > 1$. If the system is initially in a high viral load steady state, held there by control of the source s, then clearly the exact $\lambda = 0$ requires precisely that $b = 1$, the special setting alluded to above. With this as a starting point, all of the parameters T_0, c, N, and k can then be altered, and it is to this alteration that we now turn our attention.

The effect of a viral source elimination such as RTI (reverse transcriptase inhibitor) is to decrease k, the parameter measuring T-cell infection rate by virus. A perfect inhibitor makes $k = 0$, or $b = 0$, and so, from (1.6), τ^* decreases exponentially as $\exp{-t'/q}$; v has the additional $\exp{-t'}$ contribution (see Figure 1.9). An imperfect inhibitor of efficiency η_{RTI}, converting k to $k' = (1 - \eta_{\text{RTI}})k$, will still send the system to its uninfected virus-free origin if $b' = (1 - \eta_{\text{RTI}})b < 1$ or

$$(1 - \eta_{\text{RTI}})k < \frac{c}{NT_0}.$$

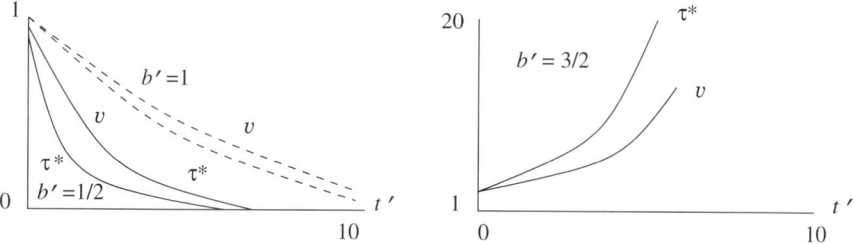

FIGURE 1.9. Time course at homeostatically stabilized T_0.

In particular, $\eta_{\mathrm{RTI}} > 0$ suffices for T_0 determined by the initial drug-free steady state, for which we know that $b = 1$. The drug fails as soon as the virus has mutated to the point that the RT inhibitor can no longer maintain this value of k' in the face of concomitant changes in c, N, and T_0.

A second category of drugs, protease inhibitors (PI), has a very different biological effect: of the N virions produced, a fraction, say $\eta_{\mathrm{PI}}N$, will be noninfectious, V_{NI}, leaving only $(1 - \eta_{\mathrm{PI}})N$ to produce the infectious V. Thus, at efficiency η_{PI}, the virus production splits into

$$\frac{dV}{dt} = (1 - \eta_{\mathrm{PI}})N\delta T^* - cV,$$

$$\frac{dV_{\mathrm{NI}}}{dt} = \eta_{\mathrm{PI}}N\delta T^* - cV_{\mathrm{NI}}.$$

But the effect on infectious virus production $V(t)$ is unchanged in form: now

$$b' = (1 - \eta_{\mathrm{PI}})\frac{NkT_0}{c},$$

and so the $b' < 1$ condition reads

$$1 - \eta_{\mathrm{PI}} < \frac{c}{NkT_0}.$$

In combination therapy, in which both RTI and PI are used, k changes as well. Thus, viral extinction requires

$$(1 - \eta_{\mathrm{PI}})(1 - \eta_{\mathrm{RTI}}) < \frac{c}{Nk\tau_0}.$$

Source Control. The parameters not yet modified are T_0 and c. Since T_0 is not really a fixed parameter but is systemically controlled by a homeostatic mechanism, we should examine how this is done. In effect, the source itself is concentration dependent, and the most reliable model for accomplishing this is a species of "logistic equation"

$$\frac{dT}{dt} = s + \xi T\left(1 - \frac{T}{T_M}\right) - dT,$$

in which T-cells are produced both by an external source—e.g., the thymus—and by replication at rate ξ, modified by repression as T approaches a control value of

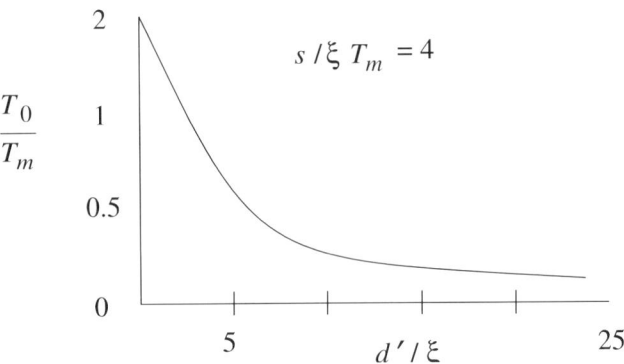

FIGURE 1.10. Viral depletion ratio.

T_M. Indeed, the population now becomes stationary, $dT/dt = 0$, at a value T_0 given by

$$(1.8) \qquad \frac{T_0}{T_M} = \pm \left[\frac{\xi - d}{\xi} + \left(\left(\frac{\xi - d}{\xi} \right)^2 + 4 \frac{s}{\xi T_M} \right)^{1/2} \right].$$

(Show that $T_0 > T_M$ or $T_0 < T_M$ as $\xi/b > T_M$ or $\xi/b < T_M$).

In the presence of virus at level V_0, the death rate d must be replaced by

$$d' = d + k V_0,$$

and we have the operating curve shown in Figure 1.10, which illustrates the basic T-cell depletion due to viral infection.

Recovery of T-cells After Initiation of Therapy. One consequence of the autonomous control is part of the recovery of T_0 seen after RTI quenches virus production. That is, suppose $T(0) = T_V$ in initial steady state, where d is replaced by the full death rate d' in the presence of virus V_0:

$$(1.9) \qquad s + (\xi - d - k V_0)T_V - \left(\frac{\xi}{T_M} \right) T_V^2 = 0.$$

Then, if V is taken as dropping to 0 at once on the scale of process considered, we have immediately after the drug treatment starts

$$\begin{aligned}
\frac{dT}{dt}\Big|_0 &= s + (\xi - d)T_V - \left(\frac{\xi}{T_M} \right) T_V^2 \\
&= k V_0 T_V.
\end{aligned}$$

Thus, after the start of therapy, T-cell levels should rise at a rate equal to the rate at which they were being infected (and killed) before therapy was initiated. It follows that the effective T_0 to be inserted into the T^* production equation is given at short time by

$$T_0(t) = (1 + k V_0 t)T_V.$$

1.4. Other Players in the Immune System

There remains the possibility of controlling the viral death rate c, and here internal interference comes into play—the normal drug-free control.

CTL Effect. We have thus far acted as if the only T-cell species of interest is the CD4 + T-cell, i.e., a T-cell with CD4 receptor, because this is the helper cell that orchestrates so much of the immune response. But there are many other cellular species that can affect the viral elimination process. We first focus on the cytotoxic T-lymphocytes (CTL)—which harbor the CD8 receptor rather than CD4—and remain available to kill antigenically marked virally infected cells, in effect increasing the viral death rate: Referring to the concentration of fully competent CTLs or effector cells as $E(t)$, and once more assuming the usual mass action chemical kinetics, the T^* and viral dynamics would now be modified to

$$(1.10) \qquad \frac{dT^*}{dt} = -(\delta + \mu E)T^* + kVT, \qquad \frac{dV}{dt} = N\delta T^* - cV.$$

Suppose that we can imagine $T = T_0$ and $E = E_0$ as held constant; then the exponents for the coupled pair of ODEs are determined as usual by

$$\det \begin{pmatrix} -\delta - \mu E_0 - \lambda & kT_0 \\ N\delta & -c - \lambda \end{pmatrix} = 0,$$

or $\lambda^2 + (\delta + c + \mu E_0)\lambda + c(\delta + \mu E_0) - N\delta kT_0 = 0$, so that the system converges to extinction at the origin if both values of $\lambda < 0$, or

$$c\left(1 + \frac{\mu}{\delta} E_0\right) > NkT_0,$$

as if we have increased the viral death rate c.

What controls the dynamics of E? Its precursors are quiescent or naive CD8 + T-cells, held homeostatically, say at L_0. These are then activated if they are simultaneously coupled to an antigen-presenting cell (APC) and a "helper" CD4 cell. Since the former should mirror the viral population, and the latter the assumedly steady population T_0, we expect that activation should occur at a rate $\zeta V T_0 L_0$ for suitable ζ. The activated CD8 + T-cells have two options, depending upon the concentration of antigenically marked cells to be targeted for destruction: they either differentiate to the lethal "effector" cells E, or they propagate and then differentiate. Any portion of the population not called upon will gradually decay. The net effect is that we can assume

$$\frac{dL}{dt} = \zeta T_0 L_0 V - \nu T^* L - \kappa L$$

for suitable decay constant κ. Finally, the net concentration of effector cells will be some multiple of the L-population entering the proliferative level but will die out at its own natural rate:

$$\frac{dE}{dt} = M\nu T^* L - d^* E.$$

At the moment, we will will simply draw the conclusion from these two equations that at steady state we will have the nontrivial relation

$$(1.11) \qquad E_0 = \left(\frac{M}{d^*}\right)\zeta T_0 L_0\left(\frac{vT^*}{\kappa + vT^*}\right)V$$

if T^* and V can be regarded as slowly varying in time, in which case $T^*(t)$ and $V(t)$ determine an $E_0(t)$.

B-Cell Interactions. CTLs prevent the birth of virus, and so decrease the excess of births over deaths, leading to an effective increase in the natural death rate c. But virus can also be neutralized and hence effectively killed on its way to infect T-cells by B-cells, the purveyors of humoral (bathing fluid) immunity. Without giving any details at this juncture, we suppose that the escape mode of the viral population, due to the virus mutating so that it is no longer recognized by the B-cells, results in a steady weakening of the B-cell lethality, and hence of the clearance rate c. Confining our attention to the consequences of this mechanism, we can ask about the slowly changing steady state in response to a slowly changing $c(t)$. Sticking to our minimal model, this means that

$$(1.12) \qquad \begin{aligned} \dot{T} &= 0 = s - dT - kVT, \\ \dot{T}^* &= 0 = kVT - \delta T^*, \\ \dot{V} &= 0 = N\delta T^* - cV, \end{aligned}$$

from which we infer that, on the high virus branch,

$$(1.12') \qquad V(t) = \frac{Ns}{c(t)} - \frac{d}{k}, \quad T(t) = \frac{c(t)}{Nk}.$$

Then indeed, a steady drop in $c(t)$ would yield a steady drop in $T(t)$, culminating in a spectacular rise in $V(t)$. Vaccine might have the opposite effect: increasing antibody, increasing c, and decreasing $V(t)$.

HIV Sanctuaries. Other cells of the immune system are CD4+ and become infected by HIV but are not destroyed as rapidly by the trauma of HIV production. For example, CD4 + macrophages are thought to emit HIV less copiously, but over a long period of time before dying, and subclasses of T-cells may do the same. Denoting the new population by M and its infected version by M^*, we would now have, in the absence of drugs,

$$\frac{dT}{dt} = s - dT - kVT,$$

$$\frac{dM}{dt} = s' - d'M - k'VM,$$

$$\frac{dT^*}{dt} = kVT - \delta T^*,$$

$$\frac{dM^*}{dt} = k'VM - \delta'M^*,$$

$$\frac{dV}{dt} = N\delta T^* + N'\delta'M^* - cV.$$

Assuming that T and M are feedback stabilized at T_0 and M_0 by augmenting the dT/dt and dM/dt equations, only the remaining three equations are relevant. In particular, steady state requires

$$T_0^* = \frac{kV_0T_0}{\delta}, \quad M_0^* = \frac{k'V_0M_0}{\delta'}, \quad \text{where } N\delta T_0^* + N'\delta'M_0^* = cV_0.$$

Note that T_0 and M_0 would therefore have to be adjusted so that

$$NkT_0 + N'k'M_0 = c.$$

But no assumptions are needed if RT and protease inhibitor therapy has started. The only new virus would then be noninfective, and we would have instead

$$\frac{dT^*}{dt} = -\delta T^*, \quad \frac{dM^*}{dt} = -\delta'M^*,$$

$$\frac{dV}{dt} = -cV, \quad \frac{dV_{\text{NI}}}{dt} = N\delta T^* + N'\delta'M^* - cV_{\text{NI}},$$

a very solvable system for which

$$T^*(t) = T^*e^{-\delta t}, \quad M^*(t) = M_0^*e^{-\delta't}, \quad V(t) = V_0e^{-ct}.$$

Consequently, $V_{\text{NI}}(t) = (d/dt + c)^{-'}(N\delta T^* + N'\delta'M^*) + Ke^{-ct}$, the sum of a particular and general solution. Since $(d/dt + c)^{-1}e^{at} = (1/a + c)e^{at}$ as a special solution, we have

$$V_{\text{NI}}(t) = \frac{N\delta}{c - \delta}T_0^*e^{-\delta t} + \frac{N'\delta'}{c - \delta'}M_0^*e^{-\delta't} + Ke^{-ct};$$

the unknown K is fixed by imposing $V_{\text{NI}}(0) = 0$. Of course, the observable virus is given by $V_{\text{tot}}(t) = V(t) + V_{\text{NI}}(t)$:

$$V_{\text{tot}}(t) = \left(V_0 - \frac{N\delta T_0^*}{c - \delta} - \frac{N'\delta'M_0^*}{c - \delta'}\right)e^{-ct}$$

$$+ \frac{N\delta}{c - \delta}T_0^*e^{-\delta t} + \frac{N'\delta'}{c - \delta'}M_0^*e^{-\delta't}.$$

The last term (δ' is by far the smallest exponent) constitutes a long-time tail, which, once the drugs are no longer effective, is released in infective form. A typical time dependence is shown in Figure 1.11.

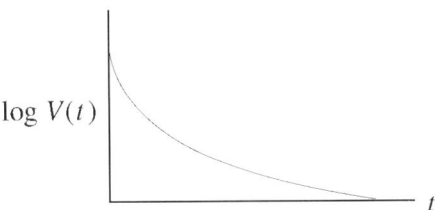

FIGURE 1.11. Generic time dependence.

1.5. Time Delay

We have more than once mentioned the possibility of time-delayed response and then ignored it. Now our ODE description by necessity chooses a few cellular and molecular types to focus on. The effect of neglected reactants is typically to buffer and delay the reaction taking place. As a trivial example, take the sequence

$$\to A \xrightarrow{k} B \xrightarrow{\ell} C$$

and imagine that B is ignored by ignorance or design. Since $\dot{C} = \ell B$, but $\dot{B} = kA - \ell B$ has the solution $B(t) = Ke^{-\ell t} + k \int_0^t A(t - t')e^{\ell t'} dt'$ (just substitute and see), then

$$\dot{C}(t) = K\ell e^{-\ell t} + k\ell \int_0^t A(t - t')e^{-\ell t'} dt'.$$

At time long compared to $1/\ell$, the K-term can be neglected and the upper limit taken to ∞, so we have

$$
\begin{aligned}
(1.13) \qquad \dot{C}(t) &= k\ell \int_0^\infty A(t - t')e^{-\ell t'} dt' \\
&\equiv k\bar{A}(t)
\end{aligned}
$$

with the interpretation that intermediate B does not change the rate $A \xrightarrow{k} C$, but all $A(t')$ for $t' < t$ contribute to $\bar{A}(t)$, albeit in decreasing weight as one goes back in time.

A much-used approximation is to replace the average memory by a single delayed amplitude. Clearly, since $A(t - t') = A(t - \tau) + (\tau - t')A'(t - \tau) + \cdots$, the first-order correction to

$$\bar{A}(t) = \ell \int_0^\infty A(t - t')e^{-\ell t'} dt' = A(t - \tau) + \left(\tau - \frac{1}{\ell}\right)A'(t - \tau) + \cdots$$

will vanish if $\tau = 1/\ell$, precisely the mean time delay:

$$\tau = \frac{\int_0^\infty t' e^{-\ell t'} dt'}{\int_0^\infty -e^{-\ell t'} dt'} = \frac{1}{\ell}.$$

We would then have

$$\dot{C}(t) = kA(t - \tau),$$

a discrete delay equation. Of course, the reverse can be carried out when a discrete time delay is realistic: it can be mimicked by a single artificial intermediary.

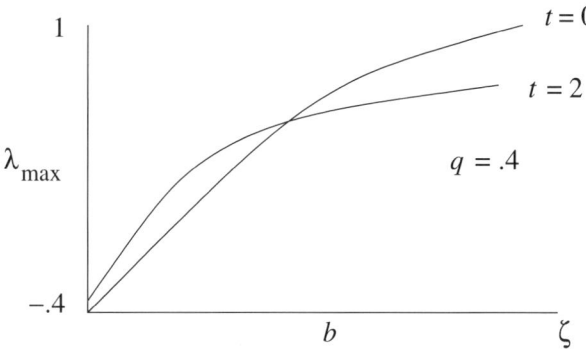

FIGURE 1.12. Decay exponent under time delay.

Delay equations introduce many novel effects, including oscillations and chaos. Let us now look only at a simple example that is devoid of such pathologies. Suppose we take into account the fact that there is certainly a time delay between the entrance of a virus into a T-cell and the exit of newly produced virions from the stricken cell. Then our basic equations (1.5) at homeostatically controlled T_0 become

(1.14)
$$\frac{dT^*(t)}{dt} = -\delta T^*(t) + kT_0V(t),$$
$$\frac{dV(t)}{dt} = N\delta T^*(t - \tau) - cV(t).$$

These are still linear homogeneous, and so we still have elementary solutions of the form $\binom{C_{T^*}}{C_V}e^{\lambda t}$. But these now imply

$$\lambda C_{T^*} = -\delta C_{T^*} + kT_0 C_V,$$
$$\lambda C_V = N\delta e^{-\lambda\tau}C_{T^*} - cC_V,$$

effectively replacing N by $Ne^{-\lambda\tau}$, or in our previously scaled notation, b by $be^{-\lambda\tau}$. Without bothering to solve the consistency equation for λ, which is changed to

(1.15)
$$q\lambda^2 + (q + 1)\lambda + 1 - be^{-\tau\lambda} = 0,$$

it is clear that precisely when $\lambda < 0$, the effect of drug therapy, which is to decrease b, is, unsurprisingly, countered by the delay (see Figure 1.12). The effect of delay will not always be unsurprising.

1.6. Conclusion

The population dynamics level of analysis we have been concerned with is highly empirical, with multiple interrelated phenomena being cartooned by a few effective parameters. It is certainly the first thing one should do in the face of wildly fluctuating incomplete data. But of course, it is knowledge of the details that enter into these model population dynamics parameters that allows nature, and ultimately allows us, to beneficially interfere with the pathological aberrations we are faced with. We now turn to these details, first in a qualitative overview, and then at a quantitative level at the many junctures in immunological response at which this is possible.

Homework Assignment 1

(1) Obtain the quoted solutions of (1.3).
(2) Derive (1.7) and its properties.
(3) Show that (1.8) has the properties cited.
(4) How does (1.12$'$) change if $c(t) = c - \alpha t$ where α is not small?

References for Chapter 1

Levine, A. *Viruses*. Scientic American Library, New York, 1992.

Perelson, A. S., and Nelson, P. W. Mathematical analysis of HIV-1 dynamics in vivo. *SIAM Rev.* 41(1): 3–44, 1999 (electronic).

CHAPTER 2

Basic Facts of Immunology

2.1. Introduction

The immune system is a complex system of cells and molecules, distributed throughout our bodies, that provides us with a basic defense against pathogens. Analogies have been drawn between the immune system and the nervous system. In fact, in primitive invertebrates (e.g., hydra), nerve cells and killer cells (nematocytes) have the same cellular progenitor, perhaps an early stage in the relationship. Like the nervous system, the immune system performs pattern recognition, learns, and remembers. The nervous system is commonly decomposed into sensory and motor parts. An analogous separation into recognition and "effector" —i.e., killing—functions is made in immunology.

The human immune system is controlled by the action of large members of *regulatory* and *effector* molecules. All the molecules that are important in the immune response have not yet been identified, but include various cell surface receptors, as well as *interleukins* that can transmit signals between cells. A variety of cell types compose the immune system, the most important being a class of white blood cells known as *lymphocytes*. These cells are transported throughout the body via the bloodstream. They can leave the blood through the capillaries, explore tissues for foreign molecules—*antigens*—or cells, and then return to the blood through the *lymph*, the fluid bathing the cells of the body. Lymphocytes spend considerable time resident in the *lymphoid organs*, such as the bone marrow, the thymus, the spleen, and lymph nodes, with small populations as well in tonsils and adenoids, small intestines, appendix, kidneys, etc. While we will dwell principally on the *acquired immunity* that results from a very sophisticated joint activity of the lymphocytes and some of their cousins, this doesn't appear immediately upon attack and constitutes a resource held in reserve. The immediate or *innate* defense is carried out by physical barriers such as the skin, chemical agents—*cytokines*— present in body fluids such as tears, and cellular police, the NK or natural killer cells.

2.2. Lymphocytes

In rough structural detail, the cells of the immune system arise in the bone marrow from the pluripotent (can produce many cellular species) *hematopoietic stem cells*, which can proliferate, or can differentiate into new stem cell progenitors of two types: white blood cell lines, either common lymphoid progenitor or myeloid progenitor; red blood cell lines, megakaryocyte or erythroblast. These events take

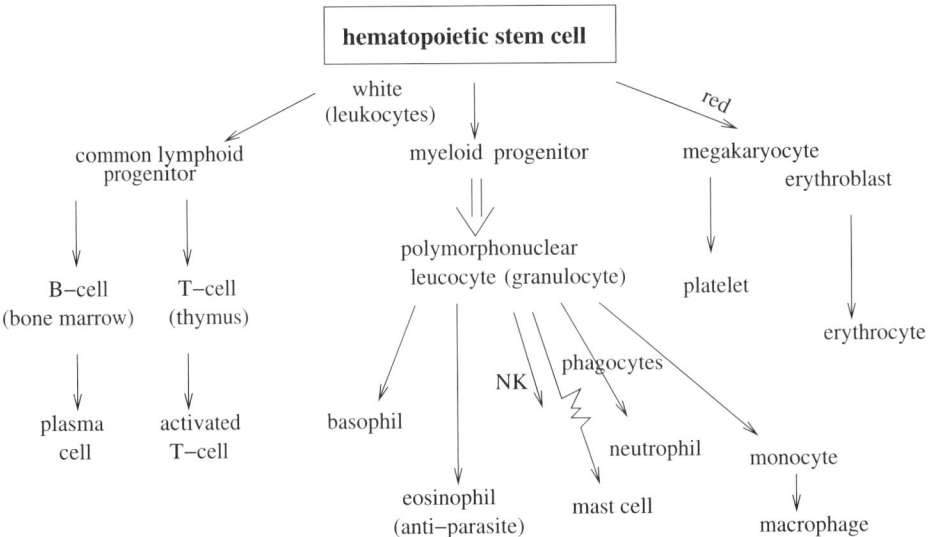

FIGURE 2.1. Family tree of major immune cell species.

place in the bone marrow, but thereafter, differentiation takes place after passage via the blood to target tissues (see Figure 2.1); however, the paths and stopovers are not known with complete confidence.

Lymphocytes are subdivided into two major classes: B-cells and T-cells. The B lymphocytes secrete *antibodies*, major protective molecules in our bodies. T-cells function mainly by interacting with other cells and have been subdivided into helper T-cells and cytotoxic T-cells. Helper T-cells, which generally express a cell surface marker called CD4, either (Th2) act through the secretion of *lymphokines* that promote the growth and differentiation of B-cells into an antibody secreting state, or (Th1, inflammatory T-cells) call macrophages into effector action. Cytotoxic T-cells, which generally express a cell surface marker called CD8, are responsible for killing virally infected cells and cells that appear abnormal, such as some tumor cells.

From the point of view of pattern recognition in the immune system, the most important feature of both B-cells and T-cells is that they have receptor molecules on their surface that can recognize antigens. In the case of B-cells, these are *immunoglobin* (antibody) molecules embedded in the membrane of the cell, but for T-cells one just speaks of the *T-cell receptors*. Recognition in the immune system occurs at the molecular level and is based upon the complementarity in shape (suitably defined) between the binding site of the receptor and an appropriate portion (or portions) of the antigen called an *epitope*. The interaction between the receptor and the epitope is not the strong chemical covalent bond, but usually involves van der Waals forces, interaction among charged groups, and hydrogen bonds. These weak interactions are nevertheless strong enough to keep the macromolecules bound when the area of interaction is sufficiently large, typically estimated as 600 Å^2.

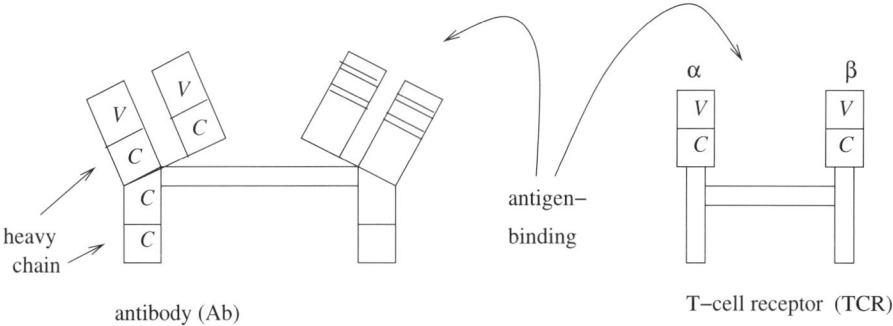

FIGURE 2.2. B- and T-cell receptors.

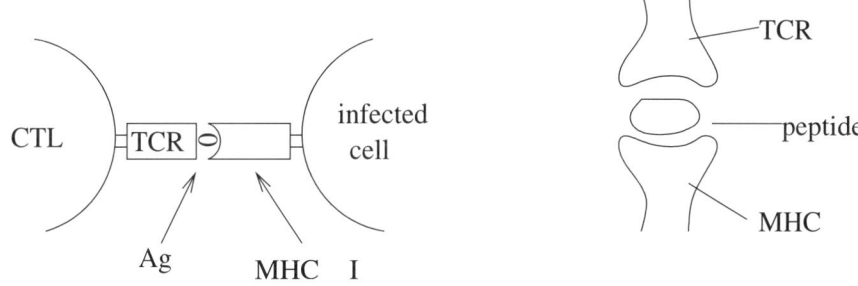

FIGURE 2.3. Signaling presence of antigen.

B- and T-cell receptors (Figure 2.2) see different features of an antigen (Ag). The B-cell receptor interacts with epitopes present on intact antigen molecules, which can be polypeptides, polysaccharides, or almost anything; these antigen molecules may be soluble or bound to a surface. The T-cell receptor only interacts with cell surface molecules, and only polypeptide. Since T-cells secrete molecules that can kill other cells or promote their growth, it is clearly important for a T-cell to "know" that it is interacting with another cell rather than with a soluble molecule. Evolution has solved this identification process by requiring the T-cell receptor to recognize omnipresent cell surface molecules known as MHC (*major histocompatibility complex*) molecules.

2.3. MHC Interactions

There are two major classes of MHC molecules, called MHC class I and MHC class II. Class I molecules are found on every cell, while class II molecules are found only on a subset of cells called *antigen-presenting cells* (APC), predominantly B-cells, macrophages, and *dendritic cells* (with a multi-arm Shiva-like appearance). Now CD8 cells—the killer T-cells—recognize MHC class I when coupled to antigen, and so start to degrade infected cells of all kinds. This requires MHC I molecules within a cell to bind peptides produced in a cell, e.g., by virus, and present them on the cell surface, which is indeed what all cells do.

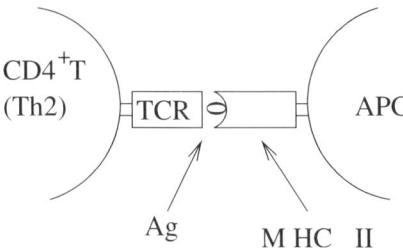

FIGURE 2.4. Role of APC.

On the other hand, APCs take up protein antigens from the environment, and partially digest them into peptides, which are transported to the surface by MHC II. The Ag–MHC II combination is recognized by CD4 helper T's, which are thereby activated and communicate with the appropriate B-cells (Figure 2.4). Lastly, in-flammatory (Th1) T-cells also recognize Ag–MHC II and call macrophages to disable the Ag-carrier. B-cells do the same by secreting Ab that tags Ag, and macrophages, recognizing this combination, start the lethal *complement cascade* (see later). Actually, complete coating of the Ag by Ab (*opsonization*) is sufficient to inactivate it, and even the binding of Ag to Ab (*neutralization*) can prevent the Ag vehicle from infecting a cell.

2.4. Receptors

Each lymphocyte has on its surface 10^4–10^5 receptor molecules, all of the same shape, that can detect antigen. There are some 10^8 B-lymphocytes and 10^8 T-lymphocytes (in the mouse) available to present different shapes to best bind the antigen, and a minimal population of ~ 10 cells seems necessary to maintain any of these lines. So only $\sim 10^7$ shapes are actually present to afford protection against the 10^{16} or so antigen types that one might be expected to encounter; all of this is a bit nebulous, depending upon how closely two shapes have to match to bind sufficiently. Now the number of possible receptor types that B-cells can genetically maintain and express is estimated as 10^{11}, with 10^{16} for T-cells, so the question is how to get to these, or even improve them. The B-cell receptor, an *immunoglob-ulin* (Ig) shown in Figure 2.2, has a structure built for this purpose: to start with, there are the *heavy-chain constant regions* (C) determining five *isotypes*: *IgA* (in body fluids), *IgM* (a pentamer—the others tend to be dimers) that can activate the complement system, *IgE* on most cells and basophils (important in inflamma-tory response and allergy), *IgD* as membrane receptor only, and *IgC* (monomer or dimer) most every place. The Ig's can be membrane bound or secreted, and the two forms are slightly different.

But the Ag-binding is due to the *variable regions* (V) derived from gene seg-ments that are inherited in a mix-or-match fashion. This is the way that B's or T's obtain their enormous repertoire. Since only $\sim 10^7$ receptor shapes can be present simultaneously, some mechanism is required to make the changes needed to con-vert the closest of the 10^7 to the Ag target to a really tight fit, measured by *affinity*.

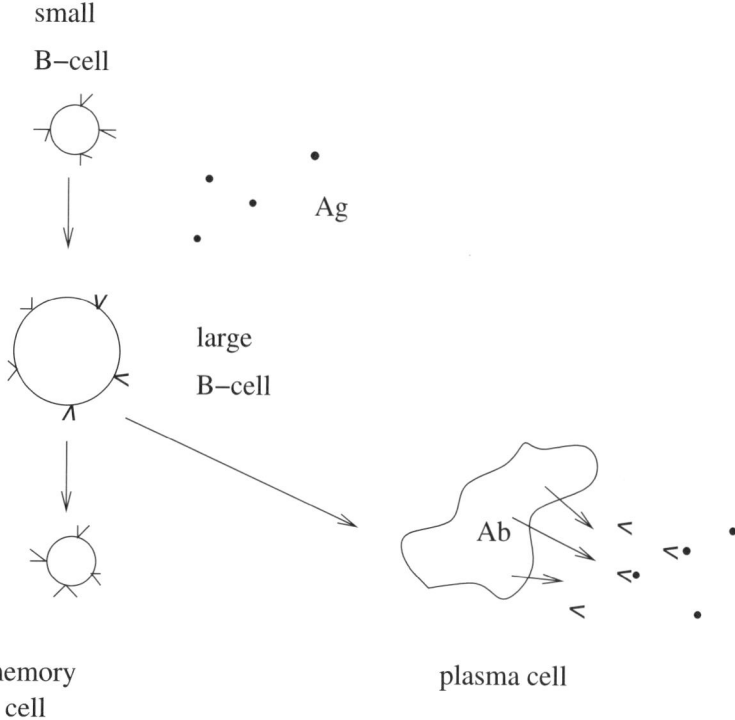

small

B−cell

Ag

large

B−cell

Ab

memory
cell

plasma cell

FIGURE 2.5. B-cell development.

This is the process of *somatic hypermutation*, leading to *affinity maturation*, in which a weakly activated cell will still proliferate, but with intentionally poor fidelity, producing a polymutant population. Mutants that bind Ag better will then reproduce faster, and the others die out, resulting in a rapid shift to a *clone* (genetically identical progeny of a single cell) of tight-binding, receptor-expressing cells. These can either differentiate to produce a long-lived *memory cell* population, proliferate, or differentiate to *plasma cells* when antigen is encountered, which secrete copious antibody if B-cells or growth factor if helper T-cells (Figure 2.5). The clone of 10^1–10^4 memory cells ready to enhance future sensitivity produced by the *clonal selection* does not of course occur randomly throughout the body, or even within a lymphoid organ, but rather at developed specific physical locations whose number is determined by the concentration of antigen to be eliminated. For example, the *humoral* (body fluid) immunity provided by B-cells is confined to *germinal centers* occupying a confined volume in which affinity maturation takes place.

2.5. Learning and Memory

Let us summarize. For protection, it is not enough to only recognize antigen. The immune system must also have sufficient resources to mount an effective response against the pathogens. As in a typical predator-prey situation, the size

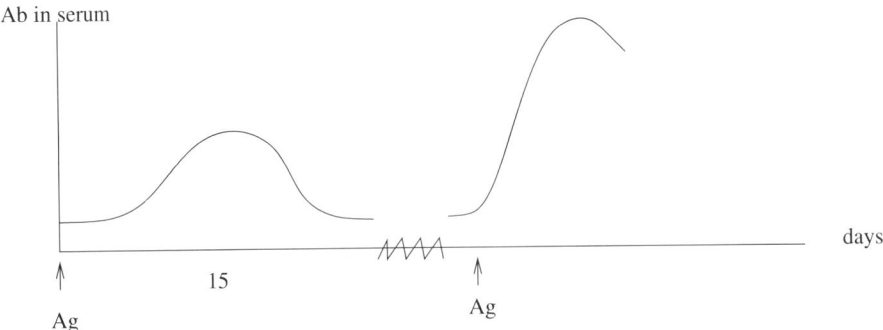

FIGURE 2.6. Primary and secondary response to Ag.

of the lymphocyte subpopulation specific for the pathogen, relative to the size of the pathogen population, is crucial in determining the outcome of infection. To be more precise, a mouse has approximately 10^8 lymphocytes. If it has a repertoire of 10^7, then on an average there are only 10 lymphocytes of any particular specificity. Learning in the immune system involves raising the population size of lymphocytes that have proven themselves to be valuable by having recognized antigen previously. If the immune system can learn from experience the shapes of antigenic *determinants* (the Ag features that are recognized), then the immune system can maintain more lymphocytes bearing receptors of the appropriate complementary shape and be better prepared to fight an antigen if it is seen again. Thus, learning in the immune system involves biasing the repertoire from random towards a repertoire that more clearly reflects the actual antigenic environment.

During the life of any individual, the detailed dynamics of lymphocyte growth, differentiation, and competition between clones ultimately reflects the system's interactionwith the environment. After an antigen has been seen once, the immune system responds to subsequent encounters with the same antigen with faster and larger amplitude responses (Figure 2.6). Such responses are called *secondary immune responses* and can be attributed to having larger initial clone sizes. Thus, say rather than starting the response with a clone of 10 cells, the system might start with 10^4 cells specific for the antigen. When these cells secrete antibody, they will have a large impact.

In primary response, there is a delay due to the fact that the cell population needs to enlarge before it can secrete substantial amounts of antibody. The more rapid and vigorous secondary response may also be due to differences between "naive" cells and cells that have seen antigen. For example, secondary response or memory cells may be easier to trigger than naive cells. Cells that have never been triggered are small and contain little cytoplasm. When triggered, they make at least 50 new proteins. One would expect many of these molecules to remain in the cell, thus making subsequent triggering events easier and faster. And of course, the affinity of antibodies for antigen may have to increase via somatic mutations that occur during the growth of lymphocyte clones. Because the total number of lymphocytes in the immune system is regulated, increases in the sizes of some clones means that other clones may have to decrease in size. The total number of lymphocytes is not kept absolutely constant. Swelling of lymph nodes, for example, allows some increase in lymphocyte populations during an immune response, but the immune system *is* a few percent of the total cells in the body, and that percentage cannot increase very much before affecting other bodily functions.

Thus, if the immune system learns only by increasing the population sizes of specific lymphocytes, it must either forget previously learned antigens, increase in size, or constantly decrease the portion of its repertoire that is generated at random and responsible for responding to novel antigens. Because of the experimental difficulties inherent in studying individual clones in vivo, it is not yet possible to decide to what degree each of these alternatives is followed.

2.6. The Self/Nonself Discrimination Problem

The repertoire of the immune system is claimed to be *complete*, meaning that it can recognize any shape. The completeness of the repertoire presents a fundamental paradox for the immune system. Because all shapes can be recognized, the immune system can recognize molecules and cells of our body as well as foreign ones. For the immune system to function properly, it needs to be able to distinguish between these two classes of molecules and cells, which are a priori indistinguishable, so as to avoid triggering an immune response against *self-antigens*, i.e., the components of our body. Not responding against self-antigen is a phenomenon called *self-tolerance*. Understanding how this is accomplished by the immune system is called the *self/nonself* discrimination problem.

The solution to the self/nonself discrimination problem is not yet at hand, but much is known. In particular, a type of clonal selection is present as T-cells first differentiate in the thymus: those T-cells that react with self-antigens have a high probability of being eliminated. The process is however incomplete, and some self-reactive T-cells are encountered outside the thymus. This can be understood since *clonal elimination* in the thymus is based on encounters between immature T-cells and self-antigens in the thymus, and presumably not all self-antigens are present in the thymus. As is often the case in biology, several mechanisms contribute to the same function, and self/nonself discrimination involves mechanisms other than thymic elimination. Much of the recent effort in theoretical immunology, as well as in experimental immunology, is devoted to the solutions of the self/nonself discrimination problem.

Homework Assignment 2

(1) One of the older HIV models is of virus V and activated T-cells T. It takes the form

$$\frac{dT}{dt} = aV - cVT, \quad \frac{dV}{dt} = gV - eVT.$$

Analyze its dynamics.

(2) Suppose that, in the reaction analyzed in (1.13), A is produced by a constant source S, and C is degraded at rate r. Check the relation between the exact solution and the various approximations.

(3) Show how (1.15) can be solved numerically by computing $\partial \lambda / \partial b$.

CHAPTER 3

Quantifying the Immune Response (Assays)

The experimental information that is the basis of immunological theory has become increasingly sophisticated with the advent of new tools, themselves immunological in concept. Ultimately, however, one still has to ask the old questions as to the size of the population of cells of various types, their rates of secretion, the concentrations of biologically active molecules, and the like.

For a population of molecules of common specificity, there are typically many molecules in a volume that is large but yet homogeneous, and the concept of concentration—molecules per unit volume—regarded as a continuous variable, becomes relevant. For example, consider the concentration of antigen conjugate to a given antibody. A prototypical estimate is via the single radial immunodiffusion techniques (SRID), in which the Ag in a compact volumeis allowed to diffuse into agar containing antiserum (antibody but no cells). Near the source, Ag is in excess and produces, for example, Ag_2Ab for divalent Ab, which is soluble and hence optically clear. At lower Ag concentration, one gets small clusters, Ag_3Ab_2, Ag_4Ab_3, ..., which are still soluble, but at low enough Ag, multisite clustering causes large complexes, and hence a light-scattering precipitating ring (Figure 3.1), to appear. The Ag concentration with this method is generally measured by comparing with standards.

Of course, many antigens can bind, at various binding energies, to a given antibody. To distinguish these, one can make use of physical characteristics, e.g., with the general class of methods lumped underthe term *immunoelectrophoresis*, in which diffusive drift under an applied electric field discriminates according to

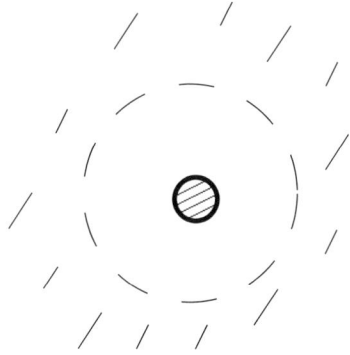

FIGURE 3.1. Reaction to dilute Ag.

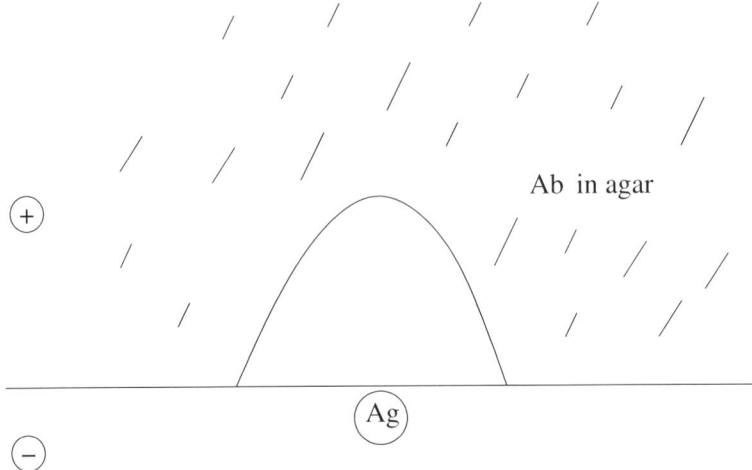

FIGURE 3.2. Rocket electrophoresis.

charge and mobility. For example, in *rocket electrophoresis*, with the geometric situation shown in Figure 3.2, the height of the precipitation arc gives a measure of the Ag concentration.

Here we will concentrate upon questions of high resolution, i.e., involving very small populations, either of cells or of the secretion from a small population of cells. For quantitative accuracy in such situations, one requires reliable mathematical control, and this will, incidentally, motivate the introduction of several mathematical techniques that will be used thereafter.

3.1. Rosette Formation

When small populations are involved, large fluctuations in any measured quantity are the norm, and probabilistic considerations become important. *Rosette formation* is an assay for the density ρ of Ab receptors on the surface of lymphocytes, macrophages, etc. The probes are the relatively small red blood cells (RBCs) whose surfaces are coated with the antibody in question, the Fc (leg) portion of which can bind, for example, to lymphocyte receptors. A number of RBCs attached to a lymphocyte, when viewed in profile, have the appearance of a rosette. Probability now enters at two different levels.

(i) First suppose that the joint area for lymphocyte-RBC adhesion is a, so that the mean number of available receptors is $\lambda = \rho a$. What is the probability of s receptors actually being present in this area? To find out, divide a into n infinitesimal areas of size Δ, so that $a = n\Delta$. The probability that a certain s of the Δ's will be occupied, $n - s$ unoccupied, is clearly $(\rho\Delta)^2(1 - \rho\Delta)^{n-s}$. Each of the s Δ's can be any of the n possible ones, and all $s!$ permutations of the order of choice give the same configuration, so the desired probability is

$$p_s = \frac{n^s(\rho\Delta)^s(1 - \rho\Delta)^{n-s}}{s!},$$

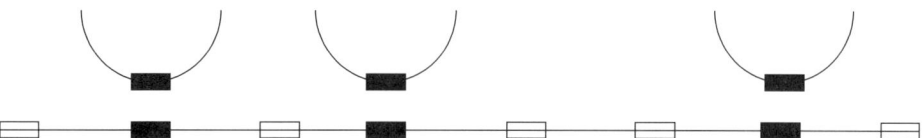

FIGURE 3.3. One-dimensional model of random sequential adsorption.

or letting $\Delta \to 0$, with $n = a/\Delta$,

$$(3.1) \qquad\qquad p_s = \frac{(\rho a)^s e^{-\rho a}}{s!}.$$

This is the *Poisson distribution* (which pops up all over the place, from the distribution of deaths due to horse kicks in the Prussian army to the number of buzz bombs hitting a London district). Now, if it takes N bound receptors for the RBC to adhere, the probability of a *given* RBC adhering is simply

$$p = \sum_{s=N}^{\infty} \frac{(\rho a)^s e^{-\rho a}}{s!}.$$

Next, what is the probability of m RBCs being bound to the cell in question? If the surface area of the cell is S, we can imagine, tentatively, that there are $M = S/a$ possible binding areas. The above argument can be repeated, but more carefully, since a is not infinitesimal. Now the number of ways that m areas out of M can be chosen to bind RBCs is just the combination coefficient

$$\binom{M}{m} = \frac{M!}{(M-m)!m!},$$

so that the associated probability is

$$P_m = \binom{M}{m} p^m (1-p)^{M-m}.$$

Finally, assuming that three or more bound RBCs are identified as a *rosette*, the relative frequency of lymphocytes appearing as rosettes should be

$$f = \sum_{m=3}^{\infty} P_m = 1 - P_0 - P_1 - P_2.$$

Given f, one can work back numerically to find ρ, and so that assay strategy is complete.

(ii) One weak point in the above is that the number M that can fit a cell is not really s/a because that would require a perfect fit, and the bound RBCs do not have the mobility to readjust. It is easier to see the problem in a one-dimensional cartoon (Figure 3.3), that of the classical "parking problem," in which cars arrive randomly and park along a curb, the number that can fit depending upon just how they arrive. In its simplest discrete version,consider a grid of extended adhesive sites in one dimension, and suppose that any cell that adheres to a site precludes the two adjacent sites from being used. There are clearly two extreme cell packings. In one extreme, they pile up as close to each other as possible, occupying every other site, for a density $n = \frac{1}{2}$. In the other extreme, gaps of two sites are left that cannot be filled, so that $n = \frac{1}{3}$. All final packings (which can accept no more cells) must then satisfy $\frac{1}{3} \leq n_\infty \leq \frac{1}{2}$. If the cells are adsorbed sequentially but randomly, what is the mean final packing density? Or equivalently the mean density of accepted sites under the restriction of next neighbor exclusion? And what is its distribution?

To solve this prototypical *random sequential adsorption* (RSA) problem, we use Flory's technique (applied originally to pair-bond formation on a polymer chain). Suppose a segment of $k > 2$ unoccupied sites, say $1, 2, \ldots, k$ with 0 and $k + 1$ occupied, has when filled to "jamming" (no cell can be added) an average of A_k vacant sites remaining. Clearly, $A_1 = 1$, $A_2 = 2$, $A_3 = 2$. But a cell dropped randomly on the unoccupied segment will adhere with equal probability $\frac{1}{k-2}$ to one of the available sites, $2, \ldots, k - 1$. If it adheres at site j, there remains one empty sublattice of $j - 1$ sites, and one of $k - j$ sites. Hence for $k > 2$,

$$(3.2) \qquad A_k = \frac{1}{k-2} \sum_{j=2}^{k-1} (A_{j-1} + A_{k-j}) = \frac{2}{k-2} \sum_{j=1}^{k-2} A_j.$$

This can be solved in many ways. Most directly, observe that

$$(k-1)A_{k+1} - (k-2)A_k = 2\left(\sum_{1}^{k-1} A_j - \sum_{j=1}^{k-2} A_j \right) = 2A_{k-1}.$$

Then, defining

$$B_k = A_{k+1} - A_k, \quad B_1 = 1, \quad B_2 = 0,$$

we have $2A_k - 2A_{k-1} = kA_{k+2} - 2(k-1)A_{k+1} + (k-2)A_k$, or

$$kB_{k+1} - (k-2)B_k - 2B_{k-1} = 0.$$

Written as

$$k(B_{k+1} - B_k) = -2(B_k - B_{k-1}) \quad \text{where } B_2 - B_1 = -1,$$

this yields at once

$$B_{k+1} - B_k = (-1)^k \frac{2^{k-1}}{k!} \quad \text{for } k \geq 1.$$

It follows that

$$B_\infty = \frac{1}{2}(1 + e^{-2}).$$

But then $n_\infty = 1 - \lim_{k \to \infty} A_k/k = 1 - \lim_{k \to \infty}(A_{k+1} - A_k) = 1 - B_\infty$, or

$$(3.3) \qquad n_\infty = \frac{1}{2}(1 - e^{-2}).$$

A little numerology is now useful. From the above, $n_\infty = .432$, which is quite close to the average $\frac{1}{2}(n_{\min} + n_{\max}) = \frac{1}{2}(\frac{1}{3} + \frac{1}{2}) = .417$. Let us proceed to a square lattice of sites with nearest-neighbor (horizontal or vertical) exclusion (see

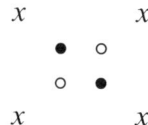

FIGURE 3.4. 2×2 sublattice; x denotes an occupied site.

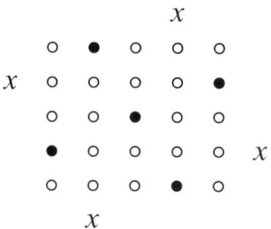

FIGURE 3.5. 5×5 sublattice; maximum final occupancy.

Figure 3.4). This cannot be solved exactly—only a few basically one-dimensional cases, discrete or continuous, can be—but numerical work gives the result

$$n_\infty = .365.$$

It is clear from a typical 2×2 cell (Figure 3.4; relevant adjacent cell occupancy shown by x) that $n_{max} = \frac{1}{2}$, and it is also clear from a typical 5×5 cell (Figure 3.5) that $n_{min} = \frac{1}{5}$. Then $\frac{1}{2}(n_{min} + n_{max}) = \frac{1}{2}(\frac{1}{5} + \frac{1}{2}) = .35$ is again a very good estimate.

This suggests that a typical jammed situation can be imagined as consisting of interwoven patches of n_{min} and n_{max}, and that a given site has equal probability of being in one or the other. It also suggests the approximation that each site independently chooses n_{min} or n_{max} (neglecting neighbor correlations, which certainly exist). Thus, quite generally, for M nominal attachment sites, the ith can be equally likely in one of two phases, specified by mean density $v_i = n_{min}$ or n_{max}. The average maximum occupancy is then

$$(3.4) \qquad \bar{M}' = \left\langle \sum v_i \right\rangle = \frac{M}{2}(n_{min} + n_{max}),$$

with a variance

$$(\delta M')^2 \equiv \left\langle \sum (v_i - \langle v_i \rangle)^2 \right\rangle = M(\langle v^2 \rangle - \langle v \rangle^2)$$

$$= M\left[\frac{1}{2}(n_{min}^2 + n_{max}^2) - \frac{1}{4}(n_{min} + n_{max})^2\right] = \frac{M}{4}(n_{max} - n_{min})^2$$

or

$$\delta M' = \frac{M^{1/2}}{2}(n_{max} - n_{min}).$$

Extending the above to what is effectively a continuum of sites on a cell surface is of course not unique, but the absolute maximum M, n_{min}, and n_{max} can all be reasonably estimated. The principal effect on the frequency f of level (i) is to replace M by $\bar{M}'$, but further corrections can be obtained by noting the quite general weak correlation expansion:

$$\langle f(M') \rangle = \langle f(\bar{M}' + (M' - \bar{M}')) \rangle$$

$$= f(\bar{M}') + f'(\bar{M}')\langle M' - \bar{M}' \rangle + \frac{1}{2} f''(\bar{M}')\langle (M' - \bar{M}')^2 \rangle + \cdots$$

or

$$\langle f(M') \rangle = f(\bar{M}'') + \frac{1}{2} f''(\bar{M}')\delta M'^2 + \cdots .$$

3.2. Limiting Dilution Analysis

This technique is for the purpose of rapidly determining the concentration of a solution of rare cells. It is rapid and relatively foolproof because it consists only of null experiments, those in which one merely has to say whether a sample contains at least one such cell or not . For example, to assay the size of a specific unactivated B-cell population, first get rid of everything else that one can—T, macrophages, complement, etc. Then prepare a concentrated, saturated (i.e., enough for all purposes) assay system of appropriate Ag-presenting cells and complement. The solution to be tested is now transformed by a hierarchy of dilutions, each dilution divided into N samples, and each sample exposed to the assay concentrate, which clonally expands any specified B-cell and indicates its presence by the cleared area of cells produced by the complement.

(i) For a preliminary estimate, suppose there are λ cells in the reference volume, and hence an average of $\rho\lambda$ in a ρ-diluted volume, or $\rho\lambda/N$ in each sample. According to the now-familiar Poisson distribution, the probability of no cells in a sample is $P(0) = \exp(-\rho\lambda/N)$, so that for $N(0; \rho)$ nonresponding samples at dilution ρ, we expect

$$(3.5) \qquad\qquad e^{-\rho\lambda/N} = \frac{N(0; \rho)}{N}.$$

Hence if $\ln(N(0; \rho)/N)$ is plotted against ρ and fitted by a straight line, one has

$$\frac{\lambda}{N} = -\frac{d}{d\rho} \ln\left(\frac{N(0; \rho)}{N} \right).$$

In other situations, one may, for example, require both a B-cell as well as a T-helper to be present in an interaction volume v around the B. If λ' is the mean number of T's in v, then a null result ensues if the sample has no B and/or no associated T, so that here

$$(3.6) \qquad\qquad P(0) = e^{-\lambda\rho/N} + e^{-\lambda'\rho/N} - e^{-\lambda\rho/N} e^{-\lambda'\rho/N}.$$

A "professional" treatment of the single-species problem involves setting up an "estimator" and maximizing it. Suppose one has a set of dilutions $\rho_1, \ldots \rho_s$, each broken into N samples, and the corresponding numbers of null-clone "successes" observed are $n_1, \ldots, n_s$ out of N. As estimator, we choose $P(\{n_i\}, \lambda)$, the probability of our set of observations on the assumption that λ cells are initially present. Since $\bar{n}_i = Ne^{-\lambda\rho_i/N}$, then

$$P(n_i) = \frac{1}{n_i!}(Ne^{-\lambda\rho_i/N})^{n_i} e^{-(Ne^{-\lambda\rho_i/N})},$$

from which

$$P(\{n_i\} \mid \lambda) = \prod \left(\frac{N^{n_i}}{n_i!}\right) e^{-\lambda \sum \rho_i n_i/N} e^{-N \sum e^{-\lambda\rho_i/N}};$$

λ is then chosen to maximize P.

$$-\ln P = \sum \ln\left(\frac{n_i!}{N^{n_i}}\right) + \lambda \sum \frac{\rho_i n_i}{N} + N \sum e^{-\lambda\rho_i/N}$$

is minimum if $\sum \rho_i n_i/N - \sum \rho_i e^{-\lambda\rho_i/N} = 0$, or

$$(3.7) \qquad \sum \rho_i \frac{n_i}{N} = \sum \rho_i e^{-\lambda\rho_i/N};$$

i.e., the ρ_i-weighted average of n_i/N is the same as that of $e^{-\lambda\rho_i/N}$. Numerical solution for λ is trivial.

(ii) A related question can be answered in a similar fashion. Are the activities of type-A and type-B antibodies on a known cell type independent or related? Now we use a lower concentration of cells and complement, divide into N samples, and inoculate each with mixed A and B sera. Anti-A and anti-B indicators are then used to test each sample as to A and B response–only A, only B, or neither—resulting in the numbers n_{AB}, $n_{A\bar{B}}$, $n_{\bar{A}B}$, and $n_{\bar{A}\bar{B}}$. If the actions are independent, one should have

$$\frac{n_{AB}}{N} = \frac{n_A}{N}\frac{n_B}{N} \quad \text{where } n_A = n_{AB} + n_{A\bar{B}}, \quad n_B = n_{AB} + n_{\bar{A}B}.$$

To check this, we compare the 2×2 "contingency table" of observations

$$\begin{pmatrix} n_{\bar{A}\bar{B}} & n_{\bar{A}B} \\ n_{A\bar{B}} & n_{AB} \end{pmatrix}$$

with the "expected"

$$\begin{pmatrix} N(1-\frac{n_A}{N})(1-\frac{n_B}{N}) & n_B(1-\frac{n_A}{N}) \\ n_A(1-\frac{n_B}{N}) & \frac{n_A n_B}{N} \end{pmatrix},$$

on the assumption of independence.

A standard comparison method involves the construction of the associated "chi-squared"

$$(3.8) \qquad \chi^2 = \sum_{\substack{i=A,\bar{A} \\ j=B,\bar{B}}} \frac{(n_{ij} - \langle n_{ij}\rangle)^2}{\langle n_{ij}\rangle}.$$

Reducing in the present case, one can show (using $n_{A\bar{B}} = Nn_A - n_{AB}$, etc.) to

$$\chi^2 = \frac{(n_{AB} - n_A n_B/N)^2}{(n_A n_B/N)(1 - n_A/N)(1 - n_B/N)}.$$

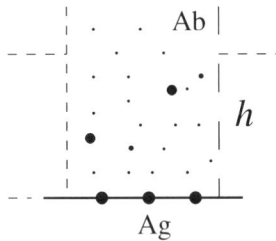

FIGURE 3.6. Model configuration of RIA and ELISA.

Now if n_A and n_B were indeed independent Poisson, this (with a little bit of work to check the denominator) would be the same $((\delta n)^2 \equiv \langle (n - \langle n \rangle)^2 \rangle = \langle n^2 \rangle - \langle n \rangle^2)$ as

$$(3.9) \qquad \chi^2 = \frac{(n_{AB} - \langle n_{AB} \rangle)^2}{(\delta n_{AB})^2}.$$

But it is well known that if n_{AB} is large enough to obey a normal distribution, the distribution of $(n_{AB} - \langle n_{AB} \rangle)/\delta n_{AB}$ would be universal, parameter independent, and hence so would be that of χ^2. If the observed χ^2 is in a low-probability region of this distribution, we would conclude dependence. Some feeling for what this region is like is supplied by the easy result that for this one-degree-of-freedom χ^2, one has

$$\langle \chi^2 \rangle = 1, \quad \delta\chi^2 = \sqrt{3}.$$

so $\chi^2 \gg 1$ certainly suggests dependence.

3.3. RIA and ELISA

Introduction. These are high-sensitivity assays for the *concentration* of Ab, which is conjugate to a given antigen. They denote *radio immuno assay* and *enzyme-linked immuno adsorbent assay*. The basic sequences in the two cases are the same:

(1) The defining antigen is bound to a plate.
(2) The Ab test solution is incubated with the plate, so that a representative concentration of Ab becomes bound to the Ag sites. The important diagnostic step in the respective assays is given by:
(3) (RIA) Concentrated Ab′, designed to bind to the Ab, is presented in radioactive form, binds to the Ab adsorbed to the plate, and the radioactivity measured.
(4) (ELISA) Similar: Ab′ is instead linked to an enzyme; on binding to the plate Ab, the enzyme activates an applied dye and so is measured.

It is in step 2 that the concentration dependence enters.

Before getting into details, let us make a quick empirical estimate of how much Ag becomes surface bound (Figure 3.6) as a function of its volume concentration. Suppose that the surface-bound antigen is characterized by the effective volume concentration $x = \text{Ag surf}/h$, the Ab solution has concentration z, and at a

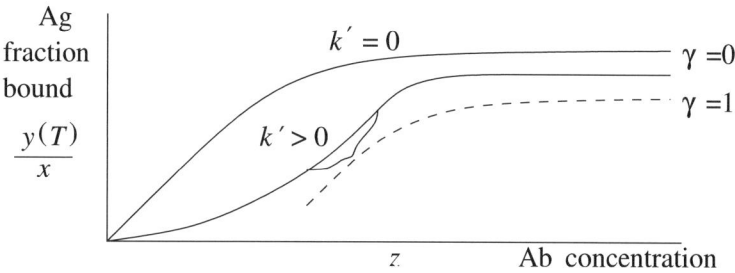

FIGURE 3.7. Dependence of Ag bound on Ab applied.

dynamic stage of the binding process, y of the antigen is bound, leaving available $x - y$ unbound antigen. If diffusion is rapid and there are many Ab molecules per Ag, the unbound Ag will be exposed to an unchanging concentration z, but if diffusion is negligible, the available mean concentration of Ab falls to $z - y$. To encompass this spectrum, we use $z - \gamma y$ for the available Ab concentration, $0 \le \gamma \le 1$:

$$\underset{z-y}{\text{Ag}} + \underset{z-\gamma y}{\text{Ab}} \underset{k'}{\overset{k}{\rightleftarrows}} \underset{y}{\text{B}}$$

Then the chemical kinetics takes the form

$$\dot{y} = k(x - y)(z - \gamma y) - k'y, \quad y(0) = 0.$$

Thus,

(1) Fast diffusion, $\gamma = 0$. $\dot{y} = kxz = (kz + k')y$, $y(0) = 0$, with the solution at time T

(3.10) $$\frac{1}{x} y(T) = \frac{kz}{kz + k'}(1 - e^{-(kz+k')T}).$$

The $k' > 0$ curve is the one observed (Figure 3.7), showing that de-adsorption is significant; the linear portion, at maximum slope, the most sensitive region, is used in practice.

(2) No diffusion, $\gamma = 1$. Now $\dot{y} = \dot{y}|_{\gamma=0} - \gamma ky(x - y)$ with a form similar to that at $\gamma = 0$.

Diffusion. If the $y - z$ curve is used to set up a calibration, everything is fine. But to predict, less hand waving is required, and the nature of spatial fluctuations enters. This brings in the quantitative nature of the diffusion process (and, on a still smaller spatial scale, that of concentration fluctuations). From the point of view of chemical kinetics, diffusion is not that strange: it is just a monomolecular interaction (Figure 3.8) between adjacent spatial compartments. For simplicity, consider a one-dimensional situation, and imagine the concentration $A(x)$ in a dx-wide interval at x, coupled to the boxes at $x - dx$ and $x + dx$, as well as to source S and sink S' at x. The chemical kinetics then reads $\dot{A}(x) = k'S - k''A(x) + kA(x + dx) + kA(x - dx) - 2kA(x)$, or Taylor-expanding $A(x \pm dx)$ to second order, simply

$$\dot{A}(x) = k'S - k''A(x) + k(dx)^2 A''(x),$$

$$S$$

$$\downarrow k'$$

$$A(x - dx) \;\overset{k}{\underset{k}{\rightleftarrows}}\; A(x) \;\overset{k}{\underset{k}{\rightleftarrows}}\; A(x + dx)$$

$$\downarrow k''$$

$$S'$$

FIGURE 3.8. Reactions equivalent to diffusion.

so defining the diffusion constant $D = k(dx)^2$, we have the *diffusion equation*

$$(3.11) \qquad \dot{A}(x) = DA''(x) - k''A(x) + k'S.$$

Generalization to three dimensions is immediate; now there are "neighbors" at $x \pm dx$, $y \pm dy$, and $z \pm dz$, and so we find at once

$$(3.12) \qquad \dot{A}(\mathbf{r}) = D\nabla^2 A(\mathbf{r}) - k''A(\mathbf{r}) + k'S.$$

For a more refined viewpoint, we can look at the component site-site net flows, e.g., from x to $x + dx$. Here there are $A(x)dx$ molecules in the interval dx around x, and $kA(x)dx$ per second are transferred to the interval about $x + dx$, of which $kA(x + dx)dx$ return. Thus, there is a positive current

$$J(x) = k(A(x) - A(x + dx))dx$$
$$= -k(dx)^2 A'(x)$$

from x; again setting $D = k(dx)^2$, this is Fick's law $J(x) = -DA'(x)$, generalizing in three dimensions to the vectorial

$$(3.13) \qquad \mathbf{J}(\mathbf{r}) = -D(\mathbf{r})\nabla A(\mathbf{r})$$

(D itself could depend upon $\mathbf{r}$). With no sources and sinks, and constant D, the diffusion equation would be equivalent to

$$(3.14) \qquad \frac{\partial A}{\partial t} + \nabla \cdot \mathbf{J} = 0,$$

the familiar particle conservation equation. Reversing the order, the diffusion equation is a consequence of Fick's law and conservation.

How does one solve the diffusion equation, say in the presence of an arbitrary source? Since any source can be built up out of a superposition of δ-functions,

$$S(\mathbf{r}, t) = \iint \delta(\mathbf{r} - \mathbf{r}')\delta(t - t')S(\mathbf{r}', t')d\mathbf{r}'\, dt,$$

and since the δ-function and its resulting concentration field can be freely translated in space and time, it is sufficient to solve for the *Green's function* satisfying

$$(3.15) \qquad \frac{\partial G(\mathbf{r}, t)}{\partial t} - D\nabla^2 G(\mathbf{r}, t) = \delta(\mathbf{r})\delta(t),$$

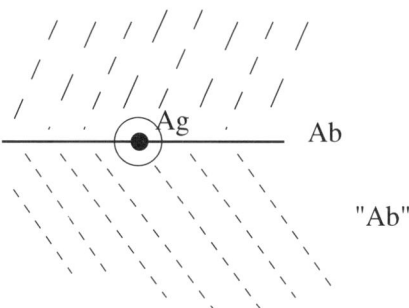

FIGURE 3.9. Full space equivalence of plane boundary.

and we can assume that $G(\mathbf{r}, t) = 0$ for $t < 0$. To obtain the solution, we take the spatial Fourier transform $\int e^{i\mathbf{k}\cdot\mathbf{r}}(\cdot)d\mathbf{r}$ over all of space. Assuming rapid vanishing at spatial infinity, one has, through integration by parts,

$$\iint (e^{i\mathbf{k}\cdot\mathbf{r}}\nabla^2 G(\mathbf{r}, t) - (\nabla^2 e^{i\mathbf{k}\cdot\mathbf{r}})G(\mathbf{r}, t))d^3 r$$

$$= \int \nabla \cdot (e^{i\mathbf{k}\cdot\mathbf{r}}\nabla G(\mathbf{r}, t) - (\nabla e^{i\mathbf{k}\cdot\mathbf{r}})G(\mathbf{r}, t))d^3 r$$

$$= \int (e^{i\mathbf{k}\cdot\mathbf{r}}\nabla G(\mathbf{r}, t) - (\nabla e^{i\mathbf{k}\cdot\mathbf{r}})G(\mathbf{r}, t)) \cdot d\mathbf{S}_\infty = 0.$$

Thus, if $g(\mathbf{k}, t) = \int G(\mathbf{r}, t)e^{i\mathbf{k}\cdot\mathbf{r}}d^3 r$, then

$$\frac{\partial g}{\partial t} + Dk^2 g = \delta(t), \quad g = 0 \text{ for } t < 0,$$

with the readily verified solution

$$g(\mathbf{k}, t) = e^{-Dk^2 t}\theta(t),$$

where θ denotes the unit step function. Now, reverse Fourier transforming

$$\left(\frac{1}{2\pi}\right)^3 \int e^{-i\mathbf{k}\cdot\mathbf{r}}(\cdot)d^3 k,$$

we conclude that

$$(3.16) \qquad G(\mathbf{r}, t) = (4\pi Dt)^{-3/2}e^{-r^2/4Dt}\theta(t),$$

and hence for an arbitrary $S(\mathbf{r}', \tau)$, with $A(\mathbf{r}, -\infty) = 0$, that

$$(3.17) \qquad A(\mathbf{r}, t) = \iint_0^t (4\pi D(t - \tau))^{-3/2}e^{-|r-r'|^2/4D(t-\tau)}S(\mathbf{r}', \tau)d\tau\, d^3 r'.$$

Time Dependence. Now we can return to the crucial step 2 of RIA and ELISA, in which Ag molecules are bound to an impenetrable substrate, so that the Ab concentration, say $c(\mathbf{r}, t)$, must have a vanishing current into the substrate. We focus on a single antigen site, imagined however as one of an ensemble of sites, and examine the full concentration field $c(\mathbf{r}, t)$. If the site is located on the substrate, the boundary condition $\hat{n} \cdot \nabla c(\mathbf{r}, t) = 0$ is satisfied automatically by completing the half-space to a full three-dimensional space (Figure 3.9). We will further give the antigen molecule spatial extension—say an impenetrable sphere of radius a. Now if $P(t)$ is the probability that the antigen has bound an Ab molecule, $Q(t) = 1 - P(t)$ for being unbound, we clearly have

$$(3.18) \qquad \dot{P}(t) = kQ(t)c(a,t) - k'P(t).$$

On the other hand, since the whole surface $4\pi a^2$ of the antigen acts as source or sink, we can write

$$\dot{c}(\mathbf{r},t) = D\nabla^2 c(\mathbf{r},t) - kQ(t)c(a,t)\frac{\delta(r-a)}{4\pi a^2} + k'P(t)\frac{\delta(r-a)}{4\pi a^2}$$
$$= D\nabla^2 c(\mathbf{r},t) - \dot{P}(t)\frac{\delta(r-a)}{4\pi a^2},$$
$$c(\mathbf{r},0) = z.$$

Solving the diffusion equation, we have

$$(3.19) \quad c(\mathbf{r},t) = z - \int_0^\infty \int (4\pi D\tau)^{-3/2} e^{-\frac{|r-r'|^2}{4D\tau}} \dot{P}(t-\tau)\frac{\delta(r'-a)}{4\pi a^2}\, d^3r'\, d\tau.$$

Defining $c(a,t) = z(t)$ and noting that

$$\int e^{-\frac{(r-r')^2}{4D\tau}}\frac{\delta(r'-a)}{4\pi a^2}\, d^3r' \bigg|_{r=a} = \int_{-1}^1 e^{-\frac{(1-\mu)}{2D\tau}a^2}\frac{1}{2}\, d\mu = \frac{D\tau}{a^2}(1 - e^{-a^2/D\tau}),$$

we conclude that

$$\dot{P}(t) = kQ(t)z(t) - k'P(t),$$
$$(3.20)$$
$$z(t) = z - \int_0^\infty \frac{(4\pi D\tau)^{-1/2}}{4\pi a^2}(1 - e^{-a^2/D\tau})\dot{P}(t-\tau)d\tau.$$

In our previous notation, $y(t) = xP(t)$, and so we recover the modified chemical kinetics

$$\dot{y}(t) = k(x - y(t))z(t) = k'y(t),$$
$$z(t) = z - \int_0^\infty \frac{(4\pi D\tau)^{-1/2}}{4\pi a^2 x}(1 - e^{-a^2/D\tau})\dot{y}(t-\tau)d\tau$$
$$= z - \gamma y(t),$$

where γ is not a number but rather the convolution operator

$$(3.21) \qquad \gamma f(t) = \int_{-\infty}^t \frac{(4\pi D(t-\tau))^{-1/2}}{4\pi a^2 x}(1 - e^{-\frac{a^2}{D(t-\tau)}})\frac{\partial}{\partial\tau} f(\tau)d\tau.$$

3.4. Hemolytic Plaque Technique

There are many methods for determining static concentrations of antigen or immunoglobin. But activated B-cells (ABF) secrete antibody for long periods, and it is the *rate* of secretion that characterizes the system. To measure this, one has Jerne's hemolytic plaque technique, which starts with a solution of Ag-coated RBCs, dark in color. On inoculation with a dilute sample of ABFs, each ABF emits a stream of Ab, diffusing into the RBC solution and binding to the RBCs

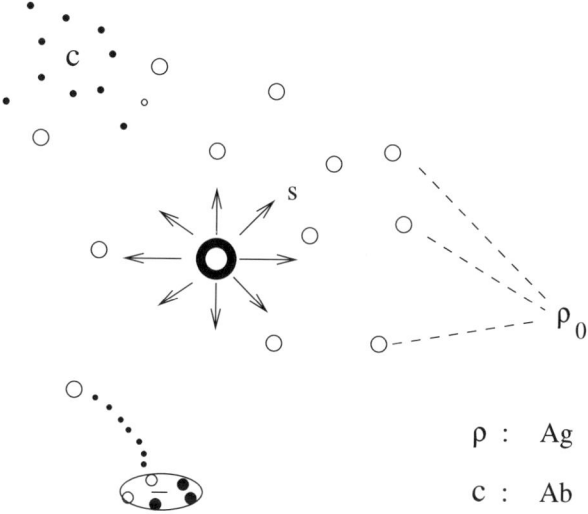

FIGURE 3.10. Hemolytic plaque formation.

at a spatially decreasing concentration whose profile moves outward in time. If complement is added, those RBCs having high enough bound Ab will be lysed, producing a colorless plaque about each ABF (Figure 3.10). The rate of plaque expansion is clearly a measure of the secretion rate. The question is, How?

Suppose that we concentrate on a single ABF at $r = 0$, secreting antibody at rate s, resulting in an inter-RBC Ab concentration $c(\mathbf{r}, t)$. Let $c_b(\mathbf{r}, t)$ be the concentration of bound Ab, the RBCs being regarded as molecules in solution for this purpose. Then in open three-dimensional space,

$$\dot{c} + \dot{c}_b = D\nabla^2 c + s\delta_3(\mathbf{r}),$$

while in a restricted space, effectively two-dimensional but of thickness h,

$$\dot{c} + \dot{c}_b = D\nabla^2 c + \frac{s}{h}\delta_2(\mathbf{r}).$$

To get a handle on c_b, if ρ_0 is the fixed nondiffusing net concentration of RBC-bound Ag, ρ the portion that is not bound to Ab, then of course

(3.22)
$$\dot{c}_b = k\rho c - k'c_b,$$
$$\rho = \rho_0 - c_b,$$

where k includes the Ab valence. Hence in local steady state, $\dot{c}_b = 0$, one has the standard Michaelis-Menten equation

$$c_b = \rho_0 \frac{Kc}{1 + Kc}, \quad K = \frac{k}{k'},$$

or assuming that $c_b \ll \rho_0$, simply

(3.23)
$$c_b = \rho_0 Kc.$$

The diffusion equation thus becomes

$$
(3.24) \qquad \dot{c} = D^* \nabla^2 c + \begin{cases} s^* \delta_3(r), & \text{3D} \\ s^*/h\delta_2(r), & \text{2D} \end{cases}
$$

where $D^* = D/(1 + K\rho_0)$, $s^* = s/(1 + K\rho_0)$.

This diffusion equation is of course again to be solved via Green's function. The two-dimensional Green's function differs from that in three dimensions by replacing the $3/2$ power by $2/2 = 1$. Since the source is now on from 0 to t, we have at once

$$
(3.25) \qquad c(r,t) = \begin{cases} s^* \int_0^t \dfrac{e^{-r^2/4D^*\tau}}{(4\pi D^*\tau)^{3/2}} \, d\tau, & \text{3D} \\ \dfrac{s^*}{4\pi h D^*} \int_0^t e^{-r^2/4D^*\tau} \, d\tau/\tau, & \text{2D.} \end{cases}
$$

Given $c(r,t)$, we can now find out how far the clear area or plaque goes. For RBC concentration ρ_{RBC} and b binding sites per RBC, we of course have $\rho_0 = b\rho_{\text{RBC}}$. Suppose that N bound Ig's are needed on an RBC to invoke lysis by complement, a binding threshold of $\bar{c}_b = N\rho_{\text{RBC}}$; since $c_b = \rho_0 K c$, we conclude that the concentration threshold $\bar{c}$ is

$$
\bar{c} = \frac{\bar{c}_b}{\rho_0 K} = \frac{N\rho_{\text{RBC}}}{\rho_0 K} = \frac{N}{bK}.
$$

The plaque then extends to distance $r(t)$ such that $c(r(t), t) = \bar{c}$. Let us estimate $r(t)$. At short time, we first rewrite our expression as

$$
(3.26) \qquad c(r,t) = \begin{cases} \dfrac{2s^*}{(4\pi)^{3/2}D^*} \dfrac{1}{r} \int_{r^2/4D^*t}^{\infty} e^{-u} du/u^{1/2}, & \text{3D} \\ \dfrac{s^*}{4\pi h D^*} \int_{r^2/4D^*t}^{\infty} e^{-u} du/u, & \text{2D,} \end{cases}
$$

and then integrate by parts,

$$
\int_u^\infty e^{-u} du/u^{1/2} = -\int_u^\infty u^{-1/2} \, de^{-u} = u^{-1/2}e^{-u} + \cdots
$$

$$
\int_u^\infty e^{-u} du/u = -\int_u^\infty u^{-1} \, de^{-u} = u^{-1}e^{-u} + \cdots
$$

to obtain at short time

$$
(3.27) \qquad \frac{r^2}{4D^*t} = \begin{cases} \ln(t^{1/2}/r^2) + \ln(s^*/2\pi^{3/2}D^{*\frac{1}{2}}\bar{c}), & \text{3D} \\ \ln(t/r^2) + \ln(s^*/\pi h\bar{c}), & \text{2D,} \end{cases}
$$

a weak dependence upon s^*. On the other hand, for long time, say in the 2D case, we use

$$
\int_u^\infty e^{-u} du/u = \int_u^\infty e^{-u} d\ln u = e^{-u}\ln u + \cdots = -\ln u + \cdots
$$

to obtain instead

$$
(3.28) \qquad \frac{r^2}{4D^*t} = e^{-4\pi h D^*\bar{c}/s^*} + \cdots, \quad \text{2D}
$$

a much stronger dependence.

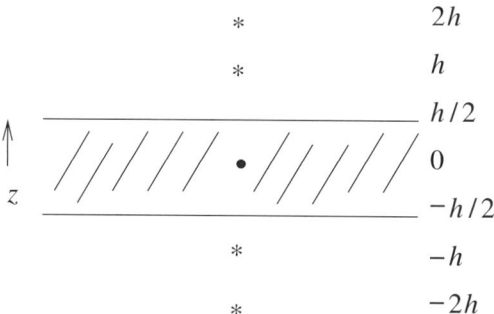

FIGURE 3.11. Simulation of slab geometry.

Clearly, the long-time regime is of major interest. But what precisely is the geometry of the system? A typical setup involves a thin slab of solution above a substrate, so we must solve the diffusion equation in a thin slab, with boundary condition of vanishing current density at $z = \pm h/2$, or $\partial c/\partial z = 0$ at $\pm h/2$. It is simplest to solve by the method of images. Assume that the point source s is at $z = 0$. If we introduce additional source *outside* the slab, the diffusion equation inside is unchanged, but if the resulting source distribution is invariant under reflection about $z = h/2$ or $-h/2$, then we will also have $\partial c/\partial z = 0$ at $z = \pm h/2$. This can be accomplished by placing virtual sources at $z = \pm h, \pm 2h, \pm 3h, \ldots$ (Figure 3.11), and hence results in a superposition of the three-dimensional solution (x denoting the two variables perpendicular to z):

$$(3.29) \qquad c(x,z,t) = s^* \int_0^t \sum_{j=-\infty}^{\infty} e^{-\frac{x^2+(z-jk)^2}{4D^*t}} \, d\tau/(4\pi D^*\tau)^{3/2}$$

(if the source is instead at $z_0 \neq 0$, we need image sources at $z_0 + 2jk$, and at $-z_0 + (2j+1)h$).

For small t, $t \ll h^2/4D^*$, then since $|z| \leq h/2$, the smallest exponent by far will be when $j = 0$, so that

$$c(x,z,t) = s^* \int_0^t e^{-(x^2+z^2)/4D^*\tau} \, d\tau/(4\pi\tau D^*)^{3/2} \quad \text{for small } t,$$

the expected span three-dimensional result, since the diffusion cloud does not yet see the surfaces. For large t, the sum converges very slowly, so that a convergence-acceleration procedure, the Poisson transformation (or θ-function transformation when applied to Gaussian sums, as here) must be introduced.

Suppose that the sum $\sum_{-\infty}^{\infty} f(j)$ converges slowly, i.e., $f(j)$ decreases slowly as $|j| \to \infty$. Then the Fourier transform

$$\tilde{f}(k) = \int_{-\infty}^{\infty} e^{iky} f(y)dy$$

will instead have a strong maximum at small k and, choosing the continuous function $f(y)$ to also have a few derivatives, will decrease rapidly in k-space. To take advantage of this, we re-express the sum in terms of the inverse transform of $\tilde{f}(k)$:

$$\sum_j f(j) = \frac{1}{2\pi} \sum_j \int_{-\infty}^{\infty} \tilde{f}(k) e^{-ijk} \, dk.$$

Now if k is an angle, $-\pi \le k \le \pi$, we know from the theory of Fourier series that $2\pi \delta(k) = \sum_j e^{-ijk}$. If k is outside $(-\pi, \pi]$, then k (mod 2π) must be used instead; thus

$$\sum_{j=-\infty}^{\infty} e^{-ijk} = 2\pi \sum_{N=-\infty}^{\infty} \delta(k - 2\pi N),$$

and the k-integration in $\sum f(j)$ yields

$$\sum_j f(j) = \sum_j \tilde{f}(2\pi N), \tag{3.30}$$

which is the Poisson formula.

In the present case,

$$f(j) = e^{-(z-jh)^2/4D^*\tau},$$

so that

$$\tilde{f}(k) = e^{-ihz/h}(4\pi D^*\tau/h^2)^{1/2} e^{-D^*\tau k^2/h^2},$$

or

$$C(xzt) = \frac{S^*}{4\pi h D^*} \int_0^t \sum_N e^{-\tau 2\pi Nz/h} e^{-D^*\tau(2\pi N)^2/h^2} e^{-x^2/4D^*\tau} \, d\tau/\tau.$$

But at long time, if $4\pi D^*t/h^2 \gg 1$, only the $N = 0$ term is significant:

$$C(xzt) = \frac{s^*}{4\pi h D^*} \int_0^t e^{-x^2/4D^*\tau} \, d\tau/\tau \quad \text{for } t \gg h^2/4\pi^2 D^*, \tag{3.30}$$

precisely the two-dimensional result, the diffusion cloud now having become uniform in the z-direction. Correction terms, for example, $N = \pm 1$, are readily applied.

Homework Assignment 3

(1) Fill in the gaps between (3.2) and (3.1), or do it your own way.
(2) Derive the "easy result" at the end of Section 2.
(3) Show how initial $A(r, o)$ can be accounted for in (3.17).
(4) Investigate the $D \to 0$ and $D \to \infty$ limits of (3.21) and compare with (3.10).
(5) In rocket electrophoresis, an electric field E is applied normal to the surface containing the Ag. The effect is to increase the normal diffusion current by σEA (A is the Ag concentration). Use reasonable assumptions to find the shape of the rocket.

References for Chapter 3

Flory, P. J. Intramolecular reaction between neighboring substitutents of vinyl polymers. *J. Amer. Chem. Soc.* 61(6): 1518–1521, 1939. doi:10.1021/ja01875a053

Goldstein, B., and Perelson, A. S. The hemolytic plaque assay: theory for finite layers. *Biophys. Chem.* 7(1): 15–32, 1977. doi:10.1016/0301-4622(77)87011-7

Lefkovits, I., and Waldmann, H. *Limiting dilution analysis of cells in the immune system*. Cambridge University Press, 1979.

Perelson, A. S. A model for antibody mediated cell aggregation: rosette formation. *Mathematics and computers in biomedical applications*, 31–37. North-Holland, Amsterdam, 1985.

CHAPTER 4

Modeling Humoral Immune Responses

4.1. Binding Process

B-lymphocytes are the heart of the humoral (body fluid) acquired immunity response. They arise as pre-B's, from hematopoetic stem cells in the bone marrow, equipped with multivalent surface IgM receptors, and then differentiate to B's, with surface IgM and IgD. Activation occurs when antigen, Ag, is bound to receptors in the presence of activated T-cells or cytokines. The B then differentiates and proliferates, yielding more B (memory) cells and (divalent) IgG secreting plasma cells. The memory cells have identical receptors on modified Ig, and respond very quickly and copiously to stimulation by the original antigen. (See Figure 4.1; c_1 denotes complement.)

The binding of two molecular species is a crucial event in all biological scenarios, and certainly in various immunological scenes. When there are multiple binding sites on one of the species, the phenomenology can be quantitatively quite different from single-site binding, and when on both, qualitatively different as well. Here we will have in mind the equilibrium state, characterized by detailed balance, i.e., balanced forward and backward reaction rates for each reaction, which will indeed be the case if there are neither loops in the reaction scheme nor external sinks that effectively provide a loop to infinity. Under these circumstances, equilibrium will indeed be achieved in time.

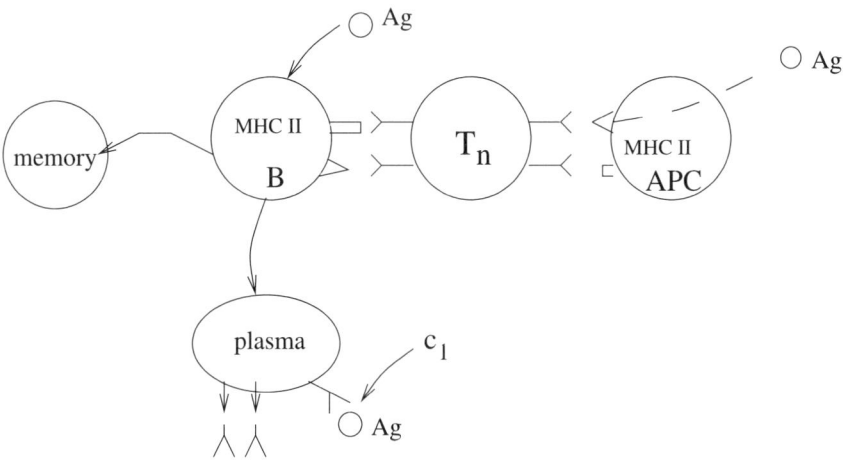

FIGURE 4.1. Events in eradication of Ag.

43

To see this, let $\{X_\alpha\}$ denote the set of reactant concentrations, and define the *Lyapunov function* (or free energy)

$$(4.1) \qquad L = \sum_\alpha X_\alpha (\ln X_\alpha / \bar{X}_\alpha - 1),$$

where $\bar{X}_\alpha$ is the equilibrium concentration belonging to X_α. Clearly, L is bounded from below,

$$(4.2) \qquad L \geq -\sum \bar{X}_\alpha \quad \text{at } \{X_\alpha = \bar{X}_\alpha\}.$$

If we can show that $dL/dt < 0$ unless $\{X_\alpha = \bar{X}_\alpha\}$, in which case $dL/dt = 0$, it will follow that $\lim_{t\to\infty} L(t) = L(0) + \int_0^\infty \dot{L}(t)dt$ converges to $L_{\min} = -\sum \bar{X}_\alpha$. Now, according to standard van't Hoff chemical kinetics, if the jth reaction causes $v_{j\alpha}$ molecules of X_α to change to $v'_{j\alpha}$ molecules for each α, then the forward and backward reaction rates are

$$(4.3) \qquad T_j = k_j \prod_\alpha X_\alpha^{v_{j\alpha}}, \quad T'_j = k'_j \prod_\alpha X_\alpha^{v'_{j\alpha}},$$

and, due to the jth reaction,

$$(4.4) \qquad \dot{X}_\beta = (T_j - T'_j)(v'_{j\beta} - v_{j\beta}).$$

Using the detailed balance assumption that $\bar{T}_j = \bar{T}'_j$ for each j, then the contribution to $\dot{L}$ of reaction j is

$$(4.5) \qquad \begin{aligned} \dot{L}_j &= (T_j - T'_j) \sum_\alpha (v'_{j\alpha} - v_{j\alpha}) \ln\left(\frac{X_\alpha}{\bar{X}_\alpha}\right) \\ &= (T_j - T'_j) \ln\left(\frac{T'_j}{T_j}\right). \end{aligned}$$

From the general relation $(a - b) \ln b/a \geq 0$ and $= 0$ only when $b = a$, we do indeed see that $dL/dt \geq 0$ and $= 0$ only when $\{X_\alpha = \bar{X}_\alpha\}$

4.2. Multivalent Binding

Affinity and Avidity. To start, imagine a well-mixed solution of Ab molecules A and antigen molecules E, with just one binding site apiece. And consider a volume with an average of one Ab molecule in a sea of fixed concentration C of antigen. If the bound pair, denoted by AE, is present at concentration x, then the chemical kinetics of the reaction

$$\underset{(1-x)}{A} + \underset{(C)}{E} \underset{k'_1}{\overset{k_1}{\rightleftarrows}} \underset{(x)}{AE}$$

(concentrations given in parentheses) reads

$$(4.6) \qquad \begin{aligned} \frac{d}{dt}(1 - x) &= k'_1 x - k_1 C(1 - x), \\ \frac{d}{dt} x &= k_1 C(1 - x) - k'_1 x. \end{aligned}$$

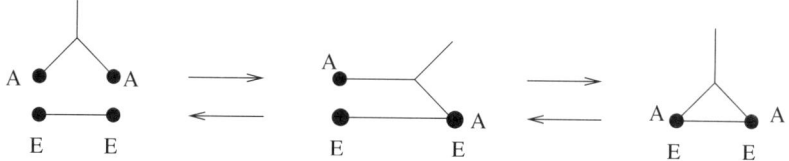

FIGURE 4.2. Genesis of avidity.

The two equations are equivalent, and in equilibrium reduce to

$$k_1(1-x)C = k_1'x.$$

Hence equilibrium is attained at

(4.7) $$x = \frac{CK_1}{1+CK_1} \quad \text{where } K_1 = \frac{k_1}{k_1'}.$$

K_1 is termed the *affinity* of the binding. An alternative form for the ratio of bound to free *ligand* (in biology, a molecule that binds to a protein) is

(4.8) $$\frac{x}{C} = K_1(1-x),$$

so that a *Scatchard plot* of x/C versus x yields K_1 as the slope.

But receptors generally have at least two sites. Why two sites? Because polymeric antigen is bound much more tightly this way: it has to come apart at *both* sites to detach. In detail, lumping the two single-bound states into one, the equilibrium kinetics of the reactions, pictured in Figure 4.2,

$$\underset{(1-x)}{AA} + \underset{(C)}{EE} \underset{k_1'}{\overset{k_1}{\rightleftarrows}} \underset{(x-y)}{A(AE)E} \underset{k_1'}{\overset{k_1}{\rightleftarrows}} (AE)^2$$

becomes $k_1(1-x)C = k_1'(x-y)$, $k_2(x-y) = k_2'y$, so that

$$y = \frac{K_2x}{1+K_2}, \quad K_1(1-x)C = \frac{x}{1+K_2}, \quad K_2 = \frac{k_2}{k_2'},$$

or

(4.9) $$x = \frac{CK_1(1+K_2)}{1+CK_1(1+K_2)},$$

an effective *avidity* (affinity for the whole multisite molecule) of

(4.10) $$K_1^* = K_1(1+K_2),$$

which can be very large indeed.

Note that in the above, the ratio $y/x = K_2/(1+K_2)$ is constant, so we may lump half-bound and fully bound together, and just refer to the binding of two composite sites, for example, one on IgM, one unit pair on the Ag. Suppose next that the Ag is a dimer, having two (composite) sites, each binding to the same Ab species. Proceeding as before, the binding sequence of Figure 4.3 becomes symbolically

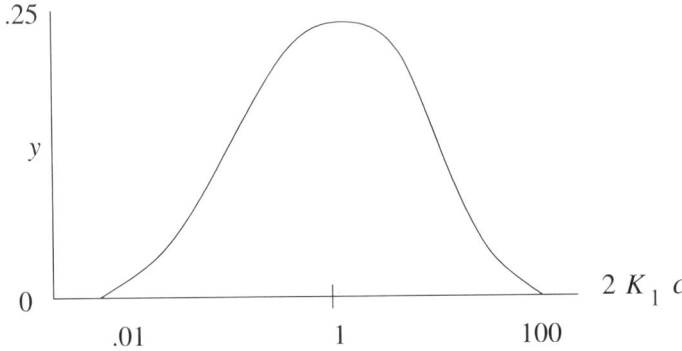

FIGURE 4.3. Two-site boundary.

FIGURE 4.4. Binding curve of Figure 4.3.

$$A + EE \underset{k_1'}{\overset{k_1}{\rightleftarrows}} A(AE)E, \qquad (AE)E + A \underset{k_2'}{\overset{k_2}{\rightleftarrows}} (AE)^2.$$
$$(1-x-2y)(C) \quad (x) \qquad\qquad (x) \quad (1-x-2y) \quad (y)$$

The equilibrium equations

$$K_1(1 - x - 2y)C = x, \qquad K_2(1 - x - 2y)x = y$$

have the solution

$$(4.11) \quad x = \beta \frac{-1 + \sqrt{1 + 4\delta}}{2\delta}, \quad y = \frac{1 + 2\delta - \sqrt{1 + 4\delta}}{4\delta},$$
$$\text{where } \beta = \frac{2K_1C}{1 + 2K_1C}, \ \delta = \beta(1 - \beta)K_2.$$

The fully bound complex (y) is now low in concentration both at low C, as expected, but at high C as well (Figure 4.4), due to the Ab being sequestered by the singly bound state. This leads to high concentration paralysis if the fully bound state is the physiologically active one, as in the analogue in which E represents complement (see later).

Let us generalize to multivalent Ag, as in a polymer or a molecular entity with similar binding sites, and imagine the Ab as mobile but surface bound. We must then specify both the valence v, the total number of accessible sites, and at least f, the mean number of accessible sites simultaneously available in a given configuration; see the example shown in Figure 4.5. For equivalent orientational configurations, we denote the concentration of all Ag states with n sites bound by C_n, the unbound Ab by S. If the bond formation rates at each stage are independent

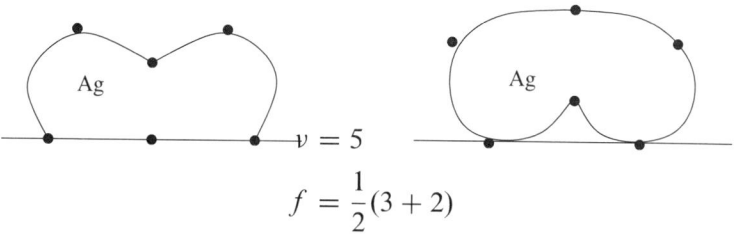

$$\nu = 5$$

$$f = \frac{1}{2}(3 + 2)$$

FIGURE 4.5. Restricted availability.

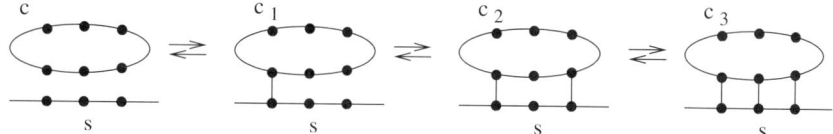

FIGURE 4.6. Multisite binding.

of bond location, the detailed balance equilibrium equations (see Figure 4.6) are

(4.12)
$$k'C_1 = k\nu CS,$$
$$k'_{i-1}iC_i = k_{i-1}(f - i + 1)C_{i-1}S, \quad i = 2, \ldots, f,$$

and antibody conservation reads

(4.12')
$$S + \sum_{1}^{f} iC_i = 1.$$

The former are solved at once as ($K = k/k'$, as usual)

$$C_1 = \nu KSC,$$

(4.13)
$$C_i = \frac{f - i + 1}{i} K_{i-1}SC_{i-1}$$
$$= \frac{\nu KC}{f} \binom{f}{i} \left(\prod_{j=1}^{i-1} K_j \right) S^i,$$

so that S is determined by

(4.14)
$$S + \nu KSC \left(1 + \sum_{i=2}^{f} \binom{f-1}{i-1} \left(\prod_{j=1}^{i-1} K_j \right) \right) S^{i-1} = 1.$$

If f depends upon the reaction channel (the orientation), these equations must be averaged.

Without loss of qualitative information, suppose that all $K_i = K'$; then

(4.15)
$$S(1 + \nu KC(1 + K'S)^{f-1}) = 1,$$

and the fully bound concentration is given by

(4.16)
$$C_f = \frac{\nu}{f} K(K')^{f-1}CS^f.$$

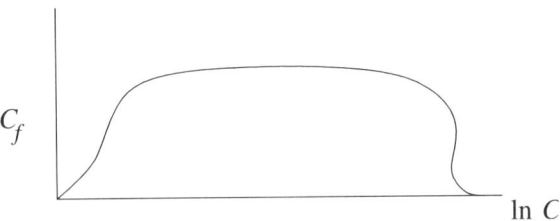

FIGURE 4.7. Double-threshold behavior.

At low concentration C, the free $S \sim 1$, and the above yields

(4.17)
$$S \sim \frac{1}{(1 + \nu K(1 + K')^{f-1}C)},$$
$$C_f \sim \frac{\nu}{f} K(K')^{f-1} \frac{C}{1 + \nu K f (1 + K')^{f-1}C}.$$

At high C, where $S \sim 0$, we have instead

(4.18)
$$S \sim \frac{1}{1 + \nu KC},$$
$$C_f \sim \frac{\nu}{f} K(K')^{f-1} e^{-\nu f KC}$$

The net effect, Figure 4.7, is an accentuated low-concentration threshold and high-concentration cutoff—a double-threshold dependence.

Homework Assignment 4

(1) The "image" method used to mimic an impenetrable barrier to diffusion in Sections 3.3 and 3.4 is convenient under many circumstances. Suppose a steady source at $(1, 1)$ in a two-dimensional layer confined to $x, y \geq 0$ (see the accompanying figure). Find the time dependence of the diffusion current at any diagonal location (R, R), and interpret.

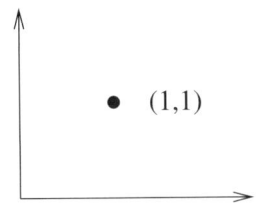

(2) The (Lotka-Volterra) reaction sequence

$$A + X \xrightarrow{k_1} 2X, \quad X + Y \xrightarrow{k_2} 2Y, \quad Y + B \xrightarrow{k_3} C,$$

at fixed concentrations A and B does *not* settle down to an equilibrium set of concentrations.

(a) Scale the kinetic equations suitably and perform a stationary point analysis.

(b) Show that $\frac{d}{dt}(f(X) + g(Y)) = 0$ for suitable f and g; what are the consequences?

(3) A reaction loop in physical space can certainly prevent equilibration. As a primitive example:

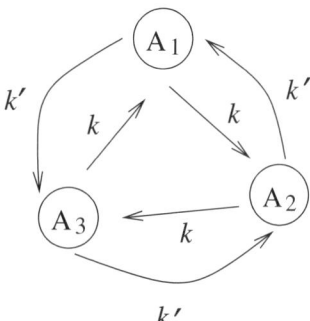

(a) Analyze the sequence shown in the accompanying figure as is.
(b) Repeat when the connection between A_3 and A_1 is broken.

4.3. Network Formation

When both components Ag and Ab are multivalent—and this is a general phenomenon—each can bind several of the other, creating a ramified *spatial* network. If this covers a significant area on a cell surface, it can have a substantial physiological effect, and it is the multivalent IgM-antigen complex (IgM has two branched receptors) that is thought to provide the signal for B-cell proliferation. In fact, one anticipates a *sol-gel* phase transition, with all molecules clustered into a single network, at a critical antigen concentration. To see how this goes, we will consider the prototype of

(4.19) bivalent Ab specified by A,
        trivalent Ag specified by E.

Physically, the network forms on the cell surface. We will neglect the possibility of spatial loops being formed—from geometric considerations, they cannot be too small—restricting ourselves to *tree* (connected but no loops) formation. And although our picture tends to be that of time development, we will ask for the nature of the equilibrium distribution of trees that results; in particular, will their mean size be arbitrarily large?

Assume an unbounded source of A at concentration S and E at concentration C. The elementary reactions are the addition of an A to an E site of a complex X:

(4.20a) $$A + X \leftrightarrows X'$$

which occurs with probability $p = KS/1 + KS$, and the corresponding addition of an E to an A site of Y:

(4.20b) $$E + Y \leftrightarrows Y',$$

with corresponding probability $p' = K'C/(1 + K'C)$. We now identify each tree

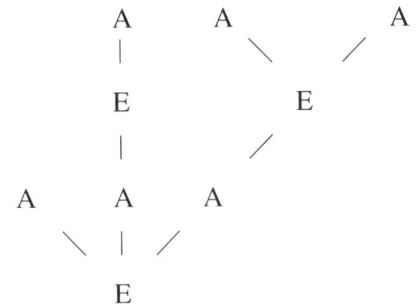

FIGURE 4.8. Development of tree network.

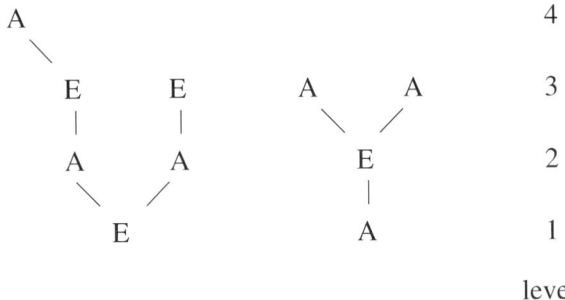

level

FIGURE 4.9. Level structure of E- and A-initiated subtrees.

solely by its components, say $A^6 E^3$ for the one shown, and weight the monomial $A^i E^j$ by $P(i, j)$, the probability of its occurrence, producing the overall description or generating function $G_E(A, E) = \sum P_E(i, j) A^i E^j$ if one starts with an E, and $G_A(A, E) = \sum P_A(i, j) A^i E^j$ if with an A. Since bonds are produced only by addition (Figure 4.8), and not within the already formed structure, in order to prevent a loop configuration, we have only to analyze the tree transformation and associated probability of occurrence for each addition to a site already present. Given an E, an A adds to it with probability p and does not add to it with probability $q = 1 - p$, so each addition corresponds to the transformation $E \to E(q + pA)$ of the generating function. An internal E can accept two A's (Figure 4.9), so

$$(4.21a) \qquad\qquad E \to E(q + pA)^2,$$

while for an initial E, $E \to E(q + pA)^3$. Similarly, E addition to an internal A performs the replacement

$$(4.21b) \qquad\qquad A \to A(q' + p'E),$$

except that $A \to A(q' + p'E)^2$ for an initial A.

To find the true asymptotic or equilibrium distribution of trees, we must carry out this process forever. To do so, we denote the full weighted sum of internal S-level, E-initiated trees by $Q_S(A, E)$, and that of S-level, A-initiated trees by $Q'_S(A, E)$. Clearly, we have

$$Q_S(A, E) = E(q + pQ'_{S-1}(A, E))^2$$

while

$$Q'_S(A, E) = A(q' + p'Q_{S-1}(A, E)).$$

Hence,

(4.22) $$Q_S(A, E) = E[q + pA(q' + p'Q_{S-2}(A, E))]^2.$$

If the process converges to Q_∞, then

(4.23) $$Q_\infty = E(q + pA(q' + p'Q_\infty))^2$$

and

$$G_A(A, E) = AQ_\infty(A, E)^2.$$

Now let us compute the mean number of A's in the network, say starting with an A. Since each term in the generating function occurs with the associated total probability, then

$$G_A(A, E) = \sum_{i,j} P_A(i, j)A^i E^j,$$

$$A\frac{\partial}{\partial A} G^A(A, E) = \sum_{i,j} iP_A(c, j)A^i E^j.$$

But $\langle n_A \rangle = \sum iP_A(i, j)$, and so we have

(4.24) $$\langle n_A \rangle = \frac{\partial G_A(A, E)}{\partial A}\bigg|_{A=E=1}$$

together, of course, with $\sum_{i,j} P_A(i, j) = 1 = G_A(1, 1)$. Directly from the equation for Q_∞,

$$\frac{\partial Q_\infty}{\partial A}\bigg|_{A=E=1}$$

$$= \bigg|q + p(q' + p'Q_\infty)^2 + 2pp'\frac{\partial Q_\infty}{\partial A}\bigg|_{A=E=1} \quad (q + p(q' + p'Q_\infty))$$

$$= 1 + 2pp'\frac{\partial Q_\infty}{\partial A}\bigg|_{A=E=1},$$

so

$$\frac{\partial Q_\infty}{\partial A}\bigg|_{A=E=1} = \frac{1}{1 - 2pp'}$$

and

(4.25) $$\langle n_A \rangle = 1 + \frac{2}{1 - 2pp'},$$

reaching a point of gelation at $pp' = \frac{1}{2}$. Similarly, for higher valence, one can show that for M_A and M_E as the mean addition rates per generation, here $2p$ and p', the gel point is at

(4.26) $$M_A M_E = 1.$$

This is utterly reasonable, since, for example, an E at one level has a mean multiplication factor $n_A n_E$ to the E's two levels forward.

The sol-gel decision need not be so direct. We have alluded to the complement cascade as a crucial endpoint in the action of acquired immunity. The cascade starts with the binding of the factor C_{1q} to surface-bound Ab and seems to require a large enough connected area of complement. Now C_{1q} is a hexamer; in early response, antibody is polyvalent IgM, and so one can imagine a gelation taking place. Later response is monomeric IgG in vast profusion. Restimulation would produce new IgM-coated cells, but now in the presence of IgG, which ought to reduce the gelation probability by competition, unless the antigenicity, and consequent IgM concentration, is high enough to justify a new attack. As a model, let E now denote trivalent complement, A divalent antibody, and B competing monovalent antibody. Singly bound E can bind A or B, bound A can bind E or B, but bound B cannot bind anything. How would the previous analysis change?

To start with, E can bind A or B; suppose the probabilities—the relative concentrations—are p and q, but now $p + q + r(\text{neither}) = 1$. Normalizing concentrations to one E-molecule, reaction balance reads

$$(4.27) \qquad \underset{(1-p-q)}{E} + \underset{(A)}{A} \underset{k'_{EA}}{\overset{k_{EA}}{\rightleftarrows}} \underset{(p)}{EA}, \quad k_{EA}(1-p-q)A = k'_{BA}p,$$

$$\underset{(1-p-q)}{E} + \underset{(B)}{B} \underset{k'_{EB}}{\overset{k_{EB}}{\rightleftarrows}} \underset{(q)}{EB}, \quad k_{EB}(1-p-q)B = k'_{EB}q,$$

solvable as

$$(4.28) \qquad p = \frac{K_{EA}A}{1 + K_{EA}A + K_{EB}B} = \frac{k_{EA}A/(1 + K_{EA}A)}{1 + \frac{k_{EB}}{K_{EA}}\frac{B}{A}\frac{K_{EA}A}{1+K_{BA}A}}$$

$$= p_0 \Big/ \left(1 + \frac{K_{EB}B}{K_{EA}A}p_0\right)$$

while

$$(4.29) \qquad q = \frac{K_{EB}}{K_{EA}}\frac{B}{A}p.$$

Similarly, A binds E or B, with probabilities p' and q', resulting in

$$(4.30) \qquad p' = p'_0 \Big/ \left(1 + \frac{K_{AB}B}{K_{AE}E}p'_0\right).$$

Now let us look at the internal trees generated from E, A, and B. They are clearly as shown in Figure 4.10, where "$-$" signifies an absent node. For S-level internal trees, we then have

$$(4.31) \qquad Q_{ES}(A, B, E) = E[pQ_{A,S-1}(A, B, E) + QB + r]^2,$$

$$Q_{AS}(A, B, E) = A[p'Q_{E,S-1}(A, B, E) + q'B + r']^2,$$

so that as $S \to \infty$, with $Q_{E\infty}(A, B, E) = Q$,

$$(4.32) \qquad Q = E[pp'AQ + pq'AB + pr'A + qB + r]^2.$$

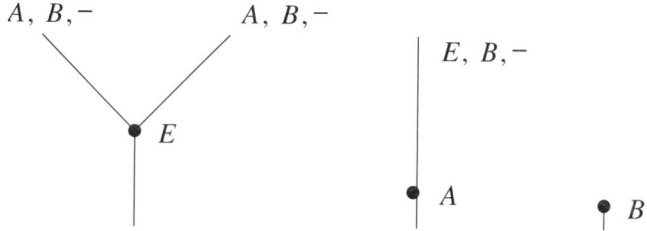

FIGURE 4.10. Elements of tree creation.

Consider the mean number of E's in an initial E-generated tree, namely,

$$\frac{\partial Q}{\partial E}\Big|_{A=B=E=1}.$$

Differentiating (4.32), $\partial Q/\partial E|_1 = 1 + 2pp'\partial Q/\partial E|_1$, whence

(4.33) $$\langle n_E \rangle = \frac{1}{1 - 2pp'},$$

as before. But p and p' don't have the same meaning. In fact, if

$$\left(\frac{K_{EB}}{K_{EA}}\right)\left(\frac{B}{A}\right) > 1,$$

then

$$p = \frac{p_0}{1 + K_{EB}B/K_{EA}A} < \frac{1}{2},$$

and no gelation can occur: the already primed system is saved from reactivating the whole complement cascade if only low Ag—as in normal cells—is present.

Homework Assignment 5

(1) Show how (4.15) and (4.16) at large f produce the extended flat portion of the $C_f - \ln C$ curve of Figure 4.7.
(2) While the mean A-population is given by (4.25), the probability of an $n_A \gg \langle n_A \rangle$ need not be negligible. Find it.
(3) In the simple analysis of (4.19), the possibility of binding loops has been explicitly discounted. Suppose that A and E can bind if $\geq s_0$ levels away. Making any necessary assumptions, determine the effect on the gelation point.

4.4. B-Cell Progression

Humoral antibody response is crucial for the detection and elimination of bacteria. A surface antigen will activate suitable small B-cells—only around 10^{-5} of the B-population will typically react to a given antigen—which then proliferates within a day or so to form a population of large B-lymphocytes. These eventually develop into memory cells with rapid strong response to the original Ag but until then, they either continue proliferating, accompanied by moderate Ab production, or differentiate into end state (unable to produce or differentiate) plasma

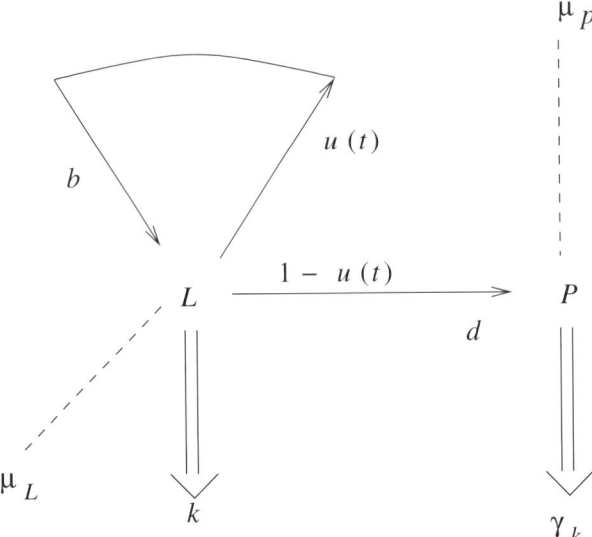

FIGURE 4.11. Short-time B-evolution.

cells which, after ~4 days, secrete copious Ab. We will first illustrate the overall evolutionary rationale behind the B-cell repertoire, and then home in on details.

Plasma-Cell Transition Control. Evolution—at the population, organism, cellular, and molecular levels, and correspondingly on an enormous range of time scales—is the driving force behind the development of present biological forms. What this means, of course, is that an entity of higher overall effectiveness in the environment that it is exposed to will eventually outreproduce and overwhelm its less fit competition. Quantitatively, characteristic parameters will evolve to optimize—maximize or minimize—appropriate figures of merit, subject in general to a variety of constraints that can, perhaps artificially (e.g., $A \geq 0 \Leftrightarrow A = z^2$) be cast as equalities. A constrained minimum (to be definite) is routinely treated by the Lagrange parameter technique, i.e., if, letting x be multidimensional, $g(x)$ is to be minimum at x_0, subject to a set of constraints $\{h_i(x) = 0\}$, $i = 1, \ldots, p$, then of course $g(x) - \sum \lambda_i h_i(x) \leq g(x_0) - \sum \lambda_i h_i(x_0)$ for any $\{\lambda_i\}$. But conversely, suppose that, given $\{\lambda_i\}$, $\{x_\lambda\}$ is found such that $g(x) - \sum \lambda_i h_i(x) \leq g(x_\lambda) - \sum \lambda_i h_i(x\lambda)$ for *all* x. Then if $\{\lambda_i\}$ is chosen so that $h_i(x_\lambda) = 0$, $i = 1, \ldots, p$, one will have $g(x) - \sum \lambda_i h_i(x) \leq g(x_\lambda)$ for all x, and consequently $g(x) \leq g(x_\lambda)$ for all x satisfying the constraints.

Now on to the short-time B-evolution context, in which we ask for the empirical repertoire of simple proliferation and end cell differentiationthat an activated B-cell population must have in order to inactivate an initial Ag load as rapidly as possible. We suppose initial exposure to an amount A^* of Ag, in antigen-antibody combining units, resulting in the production of L_0 large B-lymphocytes. At each moment, the current lymphocyte population $L(t)$ can tune the fraction $u(t)$ that reproduces at birth rate b and death rate μ_L, with Ab production at rate k. The

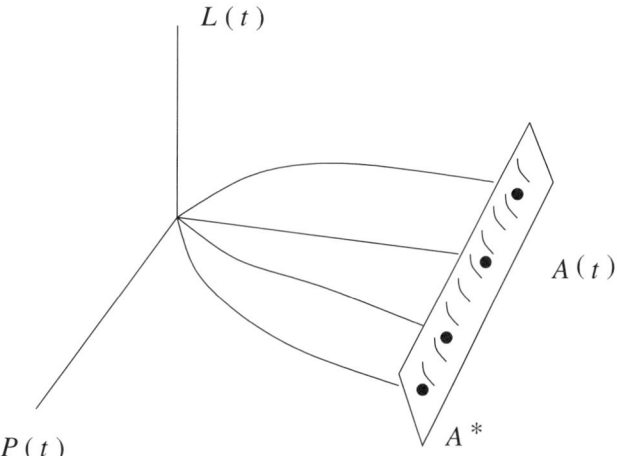

$$FIGURE\ 4.12.\ \text{System trajectories.}$$

fraction $1 - u(t)$ differentiates at rate d to P, which produces Ag at rate γk, $\gamma \gg 1$, and dies at rate μ_p. The total Ab that has been produced at time t is $A(t)$, and the elimination time T is determined by $A(T) = A^*$. We assume that $b_L \equiv b - \mu_L > 0$.

The dynamics of the system of Figures 4.11 and 4.12 is clearly given by ($\dot{x}$ denotes dx/dt)

(4.34)
$$(\dot{A}_1)\quad \dot{A} = k(L + \gamma P)$$
$$(\dot{A}_2)\quad \dot{L} = bu(t)L - d(1 - u(t))L - \mu_L L$$
$$(\dot{A}_3)\quad \dot{P} = d(1 - u(t))L - \mu_P P$$

where $A(0) = 0$, $L(0) = L_0$, and $P(0) = 0$. Producing the required neutralizing Ab in the shortest time means minimizing

(4.35)
$$J = \int_0^T dt, \quad A(T) = A^*,$$

over $\{u(t)\} \in \{U(t)\}$, where $\{0 \le U(t) \le 1\}$; $u(t)$ is allowed to be piecewise continuous to allow for sudden switches. Let us write the dynamics in the form

(4.36)
$$\dot{A}_i = f_i(\cdots A_j \cdots, u(t)), \quad i = 1, 2, 3,$$

and then introduce à la Pontryagin, Lagrange "parameters"—which now are functions—$\{\lambda_i(t)\}$ at each time to insert the dynamics in the form of subsidiary conditions. Setting $K = -\lambda_0 J$, where λ_0 will be chosen for convenience, our optimum condition becomes

Maximize over $u \in \{U\}$:

(4.37)
$$K = \int_0^T \left\{ -\lambda_0 + \sum_1^3 \lambda_i(t) \left[f_i(\cdots A_j(t) \cdots u(t)) - \dot{A}_i(t) \right] \right\} dt.$$

The dynamics (4.34) has a number of special properties that we will take advantage of. Since $u(t)$ appears undifferentiated in (4.37), we have only to select $u(t)$ to maximize.

$$(4.38) \qquad H(t) = -\lambda_0 + \sum_1^3 \lambda_i(t) f_i(\cdots A_j(t) \cdots u(t))$$

at each time, and then vary the $A_j(t)$ in (4.37). For the latter, since $\delta A_i(0) = 0$, variation of K and integration by parts yields, in general,

$$(4.39) \qquad \begin{aligned} \delta K = &-\sum \lambda_i(T)\delta A_i(T) \\ &+ \int_0^T \sum \dot{\lambda}_i(t)\delta A_i(t) + \lambda_i(t) \sum \frac{\partial f_i}{\partial A_j}(t)\delta A_j(t) dt = 0. \end{aligned}$$

Now $\delta A_1(T) = 0$, but $\delta A_2(T)$ and $\delta A_3(T)$ are arbitrary, so

$$(4.40) \qquad \lambda_2(T) = 0, \quad \lambda_3(T) = 0,$$

and we may choose λ_0 so that $\lambda_1(T) = 1$. Summarizing,

$$(4.41) \quad H(t) = \text{Max}_u, \quad \dot{\lambda}_i = -\frac{\partial(H)}{\partial A_i}, \quad \lambda_1(T) = 1, \ \lambda_2(T) = \lambda_3(T) = 0.$$

In the specific case we are studying,

$$(4.42) \qquad \begin{aligned} H = &\lambda_0 + \lambda_A K(L + \gamma P) + \lambda_L(b\mu L - d(1-u)L - \mu_L L) \\ &+ \lambda_P(d(1-w)L - \mu_P P). \end{aligned}$$

Since this is linear in the A_i, the $\dot{\lambda}_i$-equations in (4.41) can be solved without knowledge of the A_i, a great convenience. And we also observe that

$$(4.43) \qquad H = ((b+d)\lambda_L - d\lambda_P)Lu + u\text{-independent terms.}$$

But $0 \geq u \geq 1$, and so the optimal u, which we denote by u^*, has a "bang-bang control" character, i.e.,

$$(4.44) \qquad u^*(t) = \begin{cases} 1 & \text{if } \sigma(t) > 0 \\ 0 & \text{if } \sigma(t) < 0 \end{cases} \quad \text{where } \sigma(t) = (b+d)\lambda_2(t) - d\lambda_p(t),$$

and only the switch location (at most one, we will see) is in question. What we need is $\sigma(t)$. But

$$(4.45) \qquad \begin{aligned} &\dot{\lambda}_A = 0, \quad \dot{\lambda}_L = -k\lambda_A - (bu - d(1-u) - \mu_L)\lambda_L - d(1-u)\lambda_P, \\ &\dot{\lambda}_P = -\gamma k\lambda_A + \mu_P \lambda_P, \quad \lambda_A(T) = 1, \quad \lambda_L(T) = 0, \quad \lambda_P(T) = 0, \end{aligned}$$

from which

$$(4.46) \qquad \frac{1}{k}\dot{\sigma}(T) = d(\gamma - 1) - b, \quad \sigma(T) = 0,$$

to control the dynamics.

There are now two cases to consider.

Case 1. $b > d(\gamma - 1)$.

Here the large lymphocytes are sufficiently effective. In detail, we now have $\dot{\sigma}(T) < 0$ and $\sigma(T) = 0$, so $\sigma(T^-) > 0$ and $u(T^-) = 1$. Let us follow the solution back in time as long as $u(t) = 1$. During this period, we have

$$(4.47) \qquad \begin{aligned} \dot{\lambda}_P &= \mu_P \lambda_P - \gamma k, & \lambda_P(T) &= 0, \\ \dot{\lambda}_L &= -k - (b - \mu_L)\lambda_L, & \lambda_L(T) &= 0, \end{aligned}$$

which integrates back to

$$(4.48) \qquad \begin{aligned} \lambda_P(t) &= \frac{\lambda k}{\mu_P}(1 - e^{-\mu_P(T-t)}), \\ \lambda_L(t) &= \frac{\lambda k}{b_L}(e^{b_L(T-t)} - 1). \end{aligned}$$

Hence $\dot{\sigma}(t) = (b+d)\dot{\lambda}_L(t) - d\dot{\lambda}_P(t)$ tells us that

$$(4.49) \qquad \dot{\sigma}(t) = -k(b+d)e^{b_L(T-t)} + k\gamma d e^{-\mu_P(T-t)}.$$

Since $k(b+d) > \gamma d$, $e^{b_2(T-t)} > 1$, and $e^{-\mu_P(T-t)} < 1$, we have

$$(4.50) \qquad \dot{\sigma}(t) < 0,$$

and we conclude that $\sigma(t) > 0$ at all times, so that $u^*(t) = 1$ at all times.

This was the easy case.

Case 2. $b < d(\gamma - 1)$.

Hence $\sigma(T) = 0$ and $\dot{\sigma}(T) > 0$, so that $\sigma(T^-) < 0$. Now, follow the solution back in time until $\sigma(t^*) = 0$, and correspondingly

$$(4.51) \qquad \begin{aligned} u^* &= 0 & \text{on } (t^*, T), \\ u^* &= 1 & \text{on } (0, t^*) \end{aligned}$$

(the latter following the format of case 1).

Define $\mu_{Ld} = \mu_L + d$; then solving on (t^*, T) we readily find, including a subscript T to mirror the T-dependence,

$$(4.52) \qquad \sigma_T(t) = B_i^{-\mu_P(T-t)} + D - C_e^{-\mu_{Ld}(T-t)}$$

where

$$B = \frac{d\gamma k}{\mu_P}\left(1 + \frac{b+d}{\mu_P - \mu_{Ld}}\right), \qquad D = \frac{k}{\mu_{Ld}}\left(b + d + \frac{\gamma d}{\mu_P}b_L\right),$$

$$C = \frac{(b+d)k}{\mu_P}\left(\frac{\mu_P + \gamma d}{\mu_{Ld}} + \frac{\gamma d}{\mu_P - \mu_{Ld}}\right).$$

Since, on the optimal trajectory, we require $\sigma_{T^*}(t^*) = 0$ for a switch point, this gives us a transcendental equation for

$$(4.53) \qquad \tau^* = T^* - t^*.$$

This is not enough, and so we proceed to the interval $(0, t^*)$. Here, $u^* = 1$, and the set (4.34) is very easy to solve, yielding

$$(4.54) \qquad P(t) = 0, \quad L(t) = L_0 e^{b_L t}, \quad A(t) = \frac{kL_0}{b_L}(e^{b_L t} - 1).$$

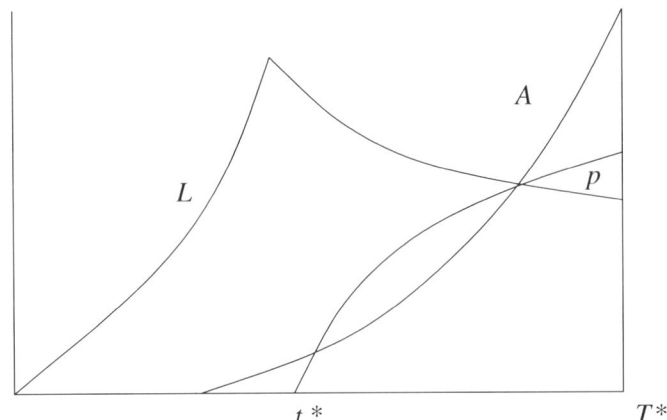

FIGURE 4.13. Dynamics of case 2.

Continuing to the interval (t^*, τ^*), where $u = 0$, we find

$$P(t) = \frac{dL_0 e^{b_L t^*}}{\mu_P - \mu_{Ld}}[e^{-\mu_{Ld}(t-t^*)} - e^{-\mu_P(t-t^*)}],$$

$$L(t) = L_0 e^{(b+d)t^* - \mu_{Ld}t},$$

(4.55)
$$A(t) = kL_0 e^{b_L t^*}\left[\frac{1}{b_L} + \frac{\mu_P + \gamma d}{\mu_{Ld}\mu_P} - \frac{(\mu_P - \mu_{Ld})t^* d}{\mu_{Ld}(\mu_P - \mu_{Ld})}e^{-\mu_{Ld}(t-t^*)}\right.$$
$$\left. + \frac{\gamma d}{\mu_P(\mu_P - \mu_{Ld})}e^{-\mu_P(t-t^*)}\right] - \frac{kL_0}{b_L}.$$

Since $A(T^*) = A^*$ and $\tau^* = T^* - t^*$ is already known, we can therefore find t^* and hence the full behavior of the system, Figure 4.13. In this case 2 regime, with the general form as indicated, we find numerically that the larger the Ag concentration A^*, the larger is the initial period of proliferation, then followed by differentiation in a bang-bang mode. Evolution indeed appears to have followed this strategy.

4.5. Evolutionary Training of Ag-Ab Complementarity

The mammalian arsenal of Ab molecules has to recognize and bind $N \sim 10^{16}$ foreign Ag's, but had better not recognize $N' < N$ self-antigens. There are "only" $n \sim 10^{11}$ antibody types constructed from permutations and combinations of an even smaller number of genetic fragments, so an Ab can only be required to match some contiguous fraction—an epitope—of an antigen molecule to maintain binding and initiate activation. How large a fraction? Perhaps quite small, say r discernible units, a unit being a number of amino acids producing a definite local configuration. We now ask how to choose r to maximize the probability P that any of the N randomly selected environmental antigens matches *at least one* of the antibodies, but none of the N' self-antigens match *any* of the n Ab's. The point is that although a successful solution of this problem will be evolutionarily maintained and strengthened by specific mechanisms that we will describe later, we have first to arrive at an adequate solution.

Let us fix the n Ab's. Let P_F be the probability that a random antigen *fails to match* a given Ab. Hence

$$\text{Pr(each of } N \text{ foreign Ag's matches at least one Ab)}$$

$$= [\text{Pr(a given foreign Ag matches at least one Ab)}]^N$$

$$= [1 - \text{Pr(a given foreign Ag matches none of the } n \text{ Ab's)}]^N$$

$$(4.56) \qquad = (1 - P_F^n)^N.$$

On the other hand,

$$(4.57) \qquad \text{Pr(none of the } N' \text{ self-antigens matches any of the } n \text{ Ab's)} = P_F^{N',n},$$

and so

$$(4.58) \qquad P = (1 - P_F^n)^N P_F^{nN'}.$$

This is maximum under selection of P_F when

$$(4.59) \qquad P_F = \left(1 + \frac{N}{N'}\right)^{-1/n} \sim 1 - \frac{1}{n} \ln\left(1 + \frac{N}{N'}\right),$$

and then

$$(4.60) \qquad P^{\max} = \left(\frac{N}{N + N'}\right)^N \left(\frac{N'}{N + N'}\right)^{N^1}.$$

Of course, $P^{\max}$ is absurdly small, so how does evolution carry out the maximization? Presumably, it does so sequentially. Suppose we define

$$(4.61) \qquad P(N, N') = \text{Pr[an Ab set can be chosen to "match" } N \text{ and } N'].$$

It is certainly reasonable to assume that

$$(4.62) \qquad \begin{aligned} &P(N, N' \mid \text{an Ab set can be chosen to match} \\ &N + \Delta N \text{ and } N' + \Delta N') = 1 \end{aligned}$$

But then from $\text{Pr}(A \mid B) = \text{Pr}(B \mid A)\,\text{Pr}(A)/\text{Pr}(B)$, we have

$$(4.63) \quad \begin{aligned} P(N + \Delta N, N' + \Delta N' \mid \text{match for } N, N') = \\ P(N + \Delta N, N' + \Delta N')/P(N, N'), \end{aligned}$$

so it is only the logarithmic increment that is to be maximized by evolution.

Imagine m types of unit with, for convenience, equal probability of occurring, and each with a complementary Ag unit. Hence, two units complement each other with a probability of $1/m$. Suppose tentatively that matching means at least r complementary pairs in sequence for two molecules, each of length ℓ and in register. Denote complementary pairs by x, noncomplementary by y, so that a pair of molecules is represented by a string of x's and y's. Failure to complement means that all contiguous x-sequences have length $< r$. To start, let us write down the generating function $G_r(x, y)$ for all non-r-matching x, y sequences of *any* length.

We do this by noting the locations of the y's and the condition that they are separated by $0, 1, \ldots, r - 1$ x's. These intervening x's are then represented by the sum $1 + x + x^2 + \cdots + x^{r-1} = (1 - x^r)/(1 - x)$. Hence

$$G_r(x, y) = \frac{1 - x^r}{1 - x} + \frac{1 - x^r}{1 - x} y \frac{1 - x^r}{1 - x} + \frac{1 - x^r}{1 - x} y \frac{1 - x^r}{1 - x} y \frac{1 - x^r}{1 - x} + \cdots$$

$$= \left(\left(\frac{1 - x^r}{1 - x} \right)^{-1} - y \right)^{-1},$$

or simply

$$(4.64) \quad G_r(x, y) = \left(\frac{1 - x}{1 - x^r} - y \right)^{-1},$$

which we note in passing is even true for x and y that do not commute, allowing for many detailed questions to be asked.

Now we can produce the generating function for comparison sequences, which are weighted by their probabilities, and by z^ℓ for length ℓ. Just let $x \to \frac{1}{m}z$, $y \to (1 - \frac{1}{m})z$, resulting in

$$G_r(z) = G_r \left(\frac{1}{m}z, \frac{m - 1}{m}z \right)$$

$$= 1 \bigg/ \left(\left(1 - \frac{1}{m}z \right) \bigg/ \left(1 - \left(\frac{1}{m} \right)^r \right) - \frac{m - 1}{m}z \right)$$

$$(4.65) \qquad = \frac{1 - (\frac{z}{m})^r}{1 - z + (m - 1)(\frac{z}{m})^{r+1}}$$

We then have to find

$$(4.66) \qquad P_F^{(\ell, r)} = \text{coef } z^\ell \quad \text{in } G_r(z),$$

and can assume that ℓ is large. One knows that if a polynomial ratio $A(z)/B(z)$ is expanded in a power series in z, then partial fractioning as

$$(4.67) \qquad \sum \frac{C_\alpha}{1 - z/z_\alpha} = \sum \frac{A(z_\alpha)/(z_\alpha B'(z_\alpha))}{1 - z/z_\alpha},$$

the high-power terms are dominated by the smallest root z^* of $B(z)$ that is not also a root of $A(z)$ (these are removable). Here then

$$(4.68) \qquad z^* = 1 + (m - 1)(z^*/m)^{r+1}.$$

For large r there is a root close to 1, and by iteration, this is given by

$$(4.69) \qquad z_1 = 1 + (m - 1)\frac{1}{m^{r+1}} + (r + 1)\left(\frac{m - 1}{m^{r+1}} \right)^2 + \cdots,$$

and, from (4.67), we conclude that for $\ell \gg r$,

$$(4.70) \qquad P_F^{(\ell, r)} = \left(1 + \frac{m - 1}{m^{r+1}} \right)^{-\ell} (1 + O(m^{-r})).$$

Now we have previously derived the requirement $P_F = (1 + N/N')^{1/n\ell}$, so it follows that

$$(4.71) \qquad 1 + \frac{m-1}{m^{r+1}} = \left(1 + \frac{N}{N'}\right)^{1/n\ell} = 1 + \frac{1}{n\ell} \ln\left(1 + \frac{N}{N'}\right) + \cdots,$$

telling us that the optimal r is given by

$$(4.72) \qquad r = \ln_m n\ell + \ln_m(m-1) - 1 - \ln_m\left(1 + \frac{N}{N'}\right) + \cdots.$$

Thus, r is essentially the total number of m-bits in n and ℓ, and consequently a quite small number, in anecdotal agreement with observation.

The model we have used can readily be dolled up—having unequal molecular lengths not in register, requiring more than one r-sequence, and so forth—but none of this changes the qualitative result.

Homework Assignment 6

(1) In a very primitive model, a macrophage progenitor M divides into two cells. Each of the two has a probability p of being another M or $q = 1 - p$ of being a macrophage end cell E, which cannot reproduce. Use generating functions to find the probability that the population is all E after N generations.

(2) An elementary version of (4.34) might simply ask for minimizing the time required to produce A^* antibody molecules when at each step one can either reproduce at rate r or effectively differentiate into a cluster of n nonreproducing Ab molecules. Solve this problem.

(3) In the evolution of Ab = Ag complementarity, estimate current $P^{\max}$ and how many generations of evolution plus consolidation would constitute a reasonable evolutionary path.

(4) How would (4.70) change if the two molecules need not be in register and in fact have different lengths ℓ_1 and ℓ_2?

4.6. Affinity Maturation

A Two-Affinity Model. Although one presumes that it is the multiepitope nature of antigens that allows them to be handled by antibodies covering sequence space of some 10–15 sites, the number of Ab types required is still much larger than the number of B-cell clones (or even B-cells) available to meet them effectively. Thus, nature has developed what might be termed a cell-cycle-length mutational strategy, so that each time weak binding and activation occur—and any B-cells carrying even lower affinity Ag will die—the following B-cell generation will have a set of "nearby" randomly mutated Ab's, some of which will bind better and thereby propagate faster. This somatic (body cells, not germ cells) hypermutation is then the basis of the process of affinity maturation, by which B-cells increase their affinity for a given antigen.

Let us start with a somewhat impressionistic version of this scheme, in which exposure to antigen (with T-cell help implied) starts the process by activating a medium affinity B-cell of a population one mutation away from high affinity. Such a cell proliferates after activation at steady rate λ, while the antigen is killing the infected organism at steady rate r. The population of interest is one mutated site, out of m relevant DNA sites, away from the high-affinity Ab, whose production neutralizes the Ag and so annuls the death rate r; we assume that the mutation rate P_n is controlled by the population size n. We want to choose the repertoire $\{P_n\}$ to minimize the probability F_1 that the initially activated system fails due to death of the host organism before settling into steady high-affinity production.

Let F_n be the probability that the system will fail in the future when it is now at population level n. The next event can either be death of the host at relative rate r, proliferation at relative rate λn, or mutation of one of the m relevant DNA sites at relative rate mnP_n. But $m-1$ of the m mutations produce a still lower affinity cell, which is eliminated from the population (one doesn't) and so we have

$$
\begin{aligned}
F_n = {} & \frac{r}{\lambda n + mnP_n + r} + \frac{\lambda n}{\lambda n + mnP_n + r} F_{n+1} \\
& + \frac{(m-1)nP_n}{\lambda n + mnP_n + r} F_{n-1}.
\end{aligned}
$$

(4.73)

We can then choose $\{P_n\}$ to minimize F_1 by imposing the "equations of motion" with Lagrange parameters, and since these equations can be written as linear in P_n, optimal strategy will again call for either $P_{\min} = 0$ or $P_{\max} = \infty$ (finite $P_{\max}$ gives similar results) at each n. There will then be one—and only one, it can be shown—switch point, say at $n = n_0$:

$$
(4.74) \qquad P_n = \begin{cases} 0 & \text{if } n \le n_0, \\ \infty & \text{if } n > n_0. \end{cases}
$$

Hence,

$$
(4.75a) \qquad n > n_0 : \quad F_n = \frac{m-1}{m} F_{n-1},
$$

$$
(4.75b) \qquad n = n_0 : \quad F_{n_0} = \frac{r}{\lambda n_0 + r} + \frac{\lambda n_0}{\lambda n_0 + r} F_{n_0+1},
$$

$$
(4.75c) \qquad n < n_0 : \quad F_n = \frac{r}{\lambda n + r} + \frac{\lambda n}{\lambda n + r} F_{n+1}.
$$

Equations (4.75a) and (4.75b) imply (take $n = n_0 + 1$)

$$
(4.76) \qquad F_{n_0} = \frac{rm}{rm + \lambda n_0},
$$

and so from (4.75a),

$$
(4.77) \qquad F_n = \left(\frac{m-1}{m} \right)^{n-n_0} \quad \text{for } n \ge n_0.
$$

Also, from (4.75c), written as

$$
(4.78) \qquad 1 - F_n = \frac{n}{n + ((r/\lambda))} (1 - F_{n+1}),
$$

we have

$$(4.79) \quad \begin{aligned} 1 - F_n &= \frac{n}{n + (r/\lambda)} \frac{n+1}{n+1+(r/\lambda)} \cdots \frac{n_0 - 1}{n_0 - 1 + (r/\lambda)} (1 - F_{n_0}) \\ &= \frac{\lambda n_0}{rm + \lambda n_0} \frac{(n_0 - 1)!}{(n-1)!} \frac{(n + (r/\lambda) - 1)!}{(n_0 + (r/\lambda) - 1)!} \quad \text{for } n \leq n_0. \end{aligned}$$

In particular,

$$(4.80) \quad F_1 = 1 - \left(\frac{r}{\lambda}\right)! \frac{\lambda n_0!}{(rm + \lambda n_0)(n_0 + (r/\lambda) - 1)!},$$

which is stationary—actually minimum—at $F_1(n_0) = F_1(n_0 - 1)$, solvable at once to yield

$$(4.81) \quad n_0 = n\left(1 - \frac{r}{\lambda}\right),$$

and correspondingly

$$(4.82) \quad F_{n_0} = \frac{mr/\lambda}{n_0 + (mr/\lambda)} = \frac{r}{\lambda}.$$

Roughly speaking, one doesn't shift from proliferation to hypermutation until each of the m closest sequences has had its chance.

4.7. Hypermutation Sequence

We have just examined a model in which the presence of antigen sets off the antibody machinery, to some extent independently of the amount of antigen present, quite the opposite of the prememory–plasma cell transition mechanism of Section 4.4. It is clearly an advantage to start the neutralization process before fine-tuning for the magnitude of antigen present, but this process itself requires much more fine-tuning than we have indicated. In particular, affinity maturation is a multistep process that can easily increase affinity by two orders of magnitude. The initial Ig (immunoglobin) is created by recombination of variable region gene segments separated by a large distance in all cells of the body except for lymphocytes. The Ig light-chain regions are built up from large V-segments and smaller J-segments (some 400 light-chain types) the heavy chains from V-, J-, and D-segments (some 10,000 heavy-chain types)—4×10^6 in all. In the presence of antigen, B-production is intentionally unreliable, and the V-segments rapidly accumulate point mutations that randomly change the binding character.

At the moment, we will say nothing of structural details, except to observe that the action takes place in a spatially confined region, so that we will often be dealing with very small populations of molecules, and the concept of concentration will not necessarily make sense. Let us start by ignoring this issue. But one we cannot ignore is that there are a large number of molecular species we may have to deal with. These are mostly simply recognized by specifying the amino acid sequence, say α, on the Ig that is going to complement the epitope—say β—on the antigen. We assume that hypermutation changes one amino acid at a time, so that the progeny of α is given by α' with the "next neighbor" property that for the jth

amino acid, $\alpha_j = \alpha'_j$ except for one mutated site; we write $\langle \alpha', \alpha \rangle$ for "α' is a next neighbor of α."

Now denote the population of B-cells by B_α of type β antigens by N_β. Then B-proliferation by N_β-binding (at fixed N_β concentration) in chemical kinetics form is

$$(4.83) \qquad B_\alpha + N_\beta \underset{k_d}{\overset{k}{\rightleftarrows}} B^*_{\alpha\beta} \overset{k_p}{\longrightarrow} 2B_\alpha$$

where

$$(4.84) \qquad \begin{aligned} \dot{B}_\alpha &= -kB_\alpha N_\beta + (2k_p + k_d)B^*_{\alpha\beta}, \\ \dot{B}^*_{\alpha\beta} &= -(k_p + k_d)B^*_{\alpha\beta} + kB_\alpha N_B, \\ \dot{N}_\beta &= -kB_\alpha N_\beta + k_d B^*_{\alpha\beta}, \end{aligned}$$

or if we assume quasi-steady state for the bound pair so that $\dot{B}^*_{\alpha\beta} = 0$, then $B^*_{\alpha\beta}$ can be eliminated, yielding

$$(4.85) \qquad \begin{aligned} \dot{B}_\alpha &= r_{\alpha\beta} B_\alpha N_\beta, \\ \dot{N}_\beta &= -r_{\alpha\beta} B_\alpha N_\beta, \end{aligned} \qquad \text{where } r_{\alpha\beta} = \frac{kk_p}{k_d + k_p}.$$

Maintaining this simplification, we then insert apoptosis of unactivated B-cells, antibody hypermutation, antigen proliferation, and possible antigen switching:

$$(4.86) \qquad \begin{aligned} \dot{B}_\alpha &= \sum_\beta r_{\alpha\beta} B_\alpha N_\beta - b(1 - h_\alpha)B_\alpha + \sum_{\langle \gamma, \alpha \rangle} \mu(B_\gamma - B_\alpha), \\ \dot{N}_\beta &= \sum_\alpha B_\alpha N_B + cN_B + \sum_{\lambda \neq \beta} \mu_{\beta\lambda} N_\lambda. \end{aligned}$$

Here

$$(4.87) \qquad h_\alpha = \frac{r_{\alpha\beta} N_\beta \Delta}{1 + \sum_\beta r_{\alpha\beta} N_\beta \Delta}, \qquad \Delta = \text{cell division time,}$$

measures the degree of activation of a clone of B-cells (after time Δ, $\sum r_{\alpha\beta} N_\beta \Delta$ new B-cells have been produced). We have neglected the role of antigen cross-linking for B-cell stimulation (which would require at least something like $B_\alpha + 2N_\beta$ in (4.83) rather than $B_\alpha + N_\beta$, as well as the role of antigen-presenting cells, and of course that of spatial heterogeneity.

One thing we should not neglect is the fact that a new B-cell species starts with a transition from population 0 to population 1 before there is any possibility of a concentration interpretation. As prototype, suppose we had a typical population ODE for particles/unit volume,

$$(4.88) \qquad \dot{x}_i = g_i(x_i) + {\sum}' m_{ji} x_i$$

in which some clones are initially unoccupied. The simplest model would say that they stay unoccupied until the predicted continuous values reach 1, and so, in the "concentration region" (4.85) would simply be replaced by

$$(4.89) \qquad \dot{x}_i = g_i(x_i)\theta(x_i - 1) + {\sum}' m_{ji} x_j \theta(x_j - 1).$$

This is what we shall do in (4.86).

Equations (4.86) are involved, even with the specializations we will make, and so we will confine our attention to numerical studies. The objective, of course, will be to find the protocol $\{\mu(t)\}$ that optimizes the binding effectiveness of the Ab population resulting after a given period of time

$$(4.90) \qquad A(T) = \sum_{\alpha\beta} B_\alpha r_{\alpha\beta}.$$

For this purpose, we can again use a version of the Pontryagin technique. In the present context, in condensed form, this would go as follows: We write the kinetic equations as

$$\dot{x}_i = g_i(x_i, \mu)x_i\theta(x_i - 1) + \sum_{j\neq i} m_{ji}(\mu)x_j\theta(x_j - 1)$$
$$= f_i(x_i\mu(t))$$

and set

$$(4.91) \qquad H((x,z;\mu(t)) = \sum_i z_i \, f_i(x;\mu(t))$$

with the $\{z_i\}$ as Lagrange parameters. The resulting equations of motion are

$$(4.92a) \qquad \dot{x}_i = \frac{\partial H}{\partial x_i} = f_i(x, \mu(t)),$$

$$(4.92b) \qquad \dot{z}_i = -\frac{\partial H}{\partial x_i} = -\sum z_j \frac{\partial f_j}{\partial x_i};$$

the terminal x-values are free to vary, but the initial values are given, and one has from the standard variational principle

$$(4.93) \qquad z_i(T) = \sum_\beta r_{i\beta}.$$

A necessary condition that $\{\mu(t)\}$ minimize $A(T)$ is that $\mu(t)$ minimize $H(t)$ pointwise for all $0 \leq t \leq T$ under the constraint $0 \leq \mu(t) \leq \mu_{\max}$. To accomplish this, we guess an initial $\{\mu_0(t)\}$ and solve (4.92a) forward in time and (4.92b) backwards in time. Then choose $\{\bar{\mu}(t)\}$ to minimize $H(\bar{\mu}(t))$ pointwise, and make the new guess

$$\mu_{n+1}(t) = \rho\mu_n(t) + (1-\rho)\bar{\mu}_n(t),$$

iterating until

$$(4.94) \qquad \frac{1}{T}\int_0^T (\mu_n(t) - \bar{\mu}_n(t))^2 \, dt < \epsilon.$$

With this numerical technique, we then find typically:

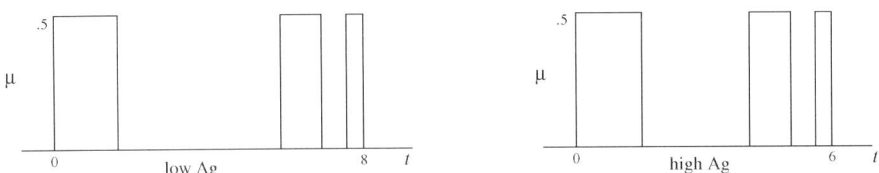

FIGURE 4.14. Optimal switching schedule.

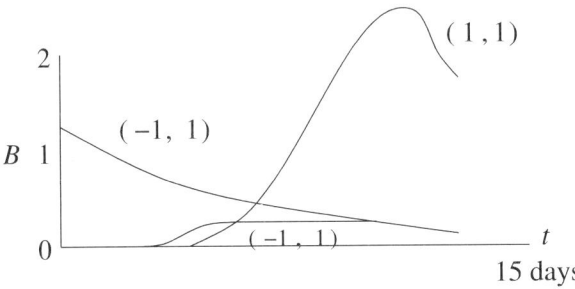

FIGURE 4.15. Dominant B-clone populations under above schedule.

Single antigen ($N_\beta = N$); $B_0 \sim 1$ cell.

$$\dot{B}_\alpha = (r_\alpha B_\alpha N - b(1 - h_\alpha)B_\alpha)\theta(B_\alpha - B_0)$$

$$+ \sum_{\langle \gamma, \alpha \rangle} (B_\gamma \theta(B_\gamma - B_0) - B_\alpha \theta(B_\alpha - B_0))$$

(4.95)

$$\dot{N} = \sum_\alpha -r_\alpha B_\alpha N \theta(B_\alpha - B_0) + cN,$$

restricted to "genome" type $\alpha = (\alpha_1, \alpha_2)$, $\alpha_i = (-1, 0, 1)$ starting with $(-1, -1)$ clone, but antigen conjugate to $(1, 1)$ alone, the others being bound weakly:
There is a dominant path $(-1, -1) \rightarrow (-1, 1) \rightarrow (1, 1)$, with other occupations negligible. Hence, expanding to a single path from a clone of $(000\ 000\ 001)$ to the high affinity $(111\ 111\ 111)$, one gets the typical phasic schedule (μ in site/cycle $\times$ 10^{-4}, t in days) shown in Figure 4.14, and the relative clone populations in Figure 4.15.

Switching antigen: The schedule is similar, but antigen escape is much easier, as it is when a continuous Ag source is present via antigen-presenting cells.

Homework Assignment 7

(1) Set up the situation expressed by (4.73) in "normal" chemical kinetic form.

(2) The quick fix of (4.88) by the strategy of (4.89) is rather crude. Consider a reaction such as

$$S \text{ (source)} \xrightarrow{k} A \xrightarrow{\ell} 2A$$

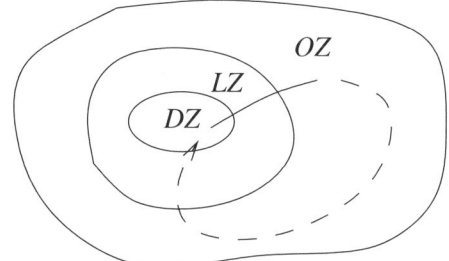

FIGURE 4.16. Activation path in germinal center.

for integer values of A, interpreting reaction rates as probabilities per unit time of reactions. Compare the result of (4.89) with the exact result.

The optimal phasic schedule must be controlled in some automatic fashion, and here the detailed spatial form is crucial. Suffice it to say that the major participant in the process is the germinal center, present in lymph nodes, the spleen, amd in other organs such as the kidney. Schematically (Figure 4.16), rapid proliferation of centroblasts takes place in the dark zone (DZ); the centroblast progeny, centrocytes, move out into the light zone (LZ), where they hypermutate and contact Ag on antigen-presenting cells, thereby being selected by affinity. They continue proliferating through the outer zone (OZ) and are thought to reenter the dark zone to restart the maturation. However, the accelerated schedule at high Ag together with the fact that the density of centers depends upon the Ag concentration, suggests that the cycle may restart in nearby centers instead (and the genetic similarity in nearby centers is similarly suggestive).

4.8. Humoral Response at Low Resolution

As our description gets more sophisticated, the coupled structure of the relevant differential equations—even the "effective concentration" regime—becomes very complex. However, the qualitative behavior of the system can often be described quite accurately in a few sentences. It would be invaluable if one could translate systematically to the low-resolution description thereby implied, and a number of techniques have been suggested for this purpose.

Let us start with an almost trivial example to illustrate both possibilities and potential difficulties. It is the Lotka-Volterra "predator-prey" system, Figure 4.17,

$$
\begin{aligned}
\dot{a} &= \lambda_1 a (h - h_0), \\
\dot{h} &= \lambda_2 h (a_0 - a),
\end{aligned}
$$
(4.96)

in which the predator a proliferates in response to excess prey $(h - h_0)$, while the prey population grows only when the predator population is sufficiently small. There are two stationary points $(a, h) = (0, 0)$ and (a_0, h_0), which are, respectively, unstable $(\delta \dot{a} = -\lambda_1 h_0 \delta a, \ \delta \dot{h} = \lambda_2 a_0 \delta h)$ and metastable $(\delta \dot{a} = \lambda_1 a \delta h, \ \delta \dot{h} = -\lambda_2 h_0 \delta a)$, the complete roster of orbits arising from the fact that

$$
K = \lambda_1 h + \lambda_2 a - \lambda_1 h_0 \ln h - \lambda_2 a_0 \ln a
$$
(4.97)

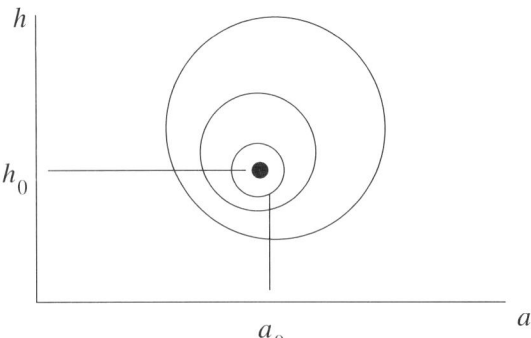

FIGURE 4.17. Predator-prey trajectories.

With (4.99) and (4.100), we can tabulate the values at $t+1$ in terms of those at t

$a(t)$	$h(t)$	$a(t+1)$	$h(t+1)$
0	0	0	1
0	1	1	1
1	0	0	0
1	1	1	0

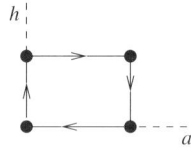

FIGURE 4.18. Discretized trajectory.

is a constant of the motion. What is clear is that this system has considerable character in its continuous domain, but the qualitative behavior is very limited. So let us construct a discrete version: $a = 0$ or 1 represents small or large a, ditto for h, t is an integer, while

$$(4.98) \qquad a(t+1) = \begin{cases} 0, & \dot{a}(t) < 0, \\ 1, & \dot{a}(t) > 0, \end{cases}$$

and ditto for h.

In this example, we must set the reference (a_0, h_0) as something intermediate, say $(\frac{1}{2}, \frac{1}{2})$, but also $\dot{a} = 0$, $\dot{h} = 0$ leads to a quandary, which we fix by replacing the original equations by

$$(4.99) \qquad \dot{a} = (a + \epsilon)(h - \tfrac{1}{2}), \quad \dot{h} = (h + \epsilon)(\tfrac{1}{2} - a),$$

corresponding to the trajectory shown, Figure 4.18. In logical notation, the one-step transformation is simply

$$(4.100) \qquad a' = h, \quad h' = \bar{a},$$

with only the trivial constant of motion $K = a(1 - a) + h(1 - h)$.

Of course, the ϵ-modification is not unique; we could equally well have written

$$(4.101) \qquad \dot{a} = (a + \epsilon)(h - \tfrac{1}{2}), \quad \dot{h} = (h - \epsilon)(\tfrac{1}{2} - a)$$

(the other two possibilities don't even cycle), and now

$a(t)$	$h(t)$	$a(t+1)$	$h(t+1)$
0	0	0	1
0	1	1	1
1	0	0	1
1	1	1	0

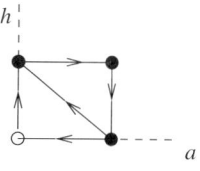

or, concisely,

$$(4.102) \qquad a' = h, \quad h' = \bar{a}h + a\bar{h},$$

with the nontrivial constant of the motion

$$(4.103) \qquad K = \bar{a}\bar{h}.$$

A further abbreviated notation is to simply place a bar over an entry that changes at the next step, so the two cases become

a	h
0	$\bar{0}$
$\bar{0}$	1
$\bar{1}$	0
1	$\bar{1}$

a	h
0	0
$\bar{0}$	1
$\bar{1}$	$\bar{0}$
1	$\bar{1}$

The utility of this construction is that it may also be used in reverse order. That is, we start with "logical structure" that represents the phenomenology, and then convert this to differential form to permit quantitative analysis. We consider an elementary example, in which species a inhibits b, which stimulates c, which inhibits a, as indicated in Figure 4.19, where inhibition is noted explicitly.

The corresponding transition table is also given in Table 4.1, together with the (redundant) next-step states—or rates—as called for in the interpretation. To turn the logical structure into a set of ODEs (the stationary, unbarred triplets have been circled), we first write out the symbolic dynamics

$$(4.104) \qquad a' = \bar{c}, \quad b' = \bar{a}, \quad c' = b,$$

and then introduce Hill-type sigmoidal stimulation and inhibition functions

$$(4.105) \qquad F_\lambda^+(x) = \frac{x^n}{\theta_\lambda^n + x^n}, \quad F_\lambda^-(x) = \frac{\theta_\lambda^n}{\theta_\lambda^n + x^n},$$

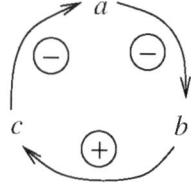

FIGURE 4.19. Prototype inhibition-stimulation network.

a	b	c	a'	b'	c'
$\bar{0}$	$\bar{0}$	0	1	1	0
0	$\bar{0}$	$\bar{1}$	0	1	0
0	1	1	0	1	1
$\bar{0}$	1	$\bar{0}$	1	1	1
1	$\bar{1}$	0	1	0	1
$\bar{1}$	$\bar{1}$	1	0	0	1
$\bar{1}$	0	$\bar{1}$	0	0	0
1	0	0	1	0	0

TABLE 4.1. Discrete transitions of Figure 4.19.

together with intrinsic decay rates, so that a species will be driven downward (rate 0) if it is not stimulated (rate 1).

The above then becomes

$$\dot{a} = kF_A^-(c) - \alpha a,$$
$$(4.106) \qquad \dot{b} = k'F_b^-(a) - \beta b,$$
$$\dot{c} = k''F_c^+(b) - \gamma c.$$

More generally, if one has, for example, a symbolic dynamics

$$(4.107) \qquad a' = a \cdot \bar{b} + c,$$

where $\cdot$ and $+$ indicate logical product (intersection) and sum (union), this might translate simply as

$$(4.108) \qquad \dot{a} = kF^+(a)F^-(b) + k'F^+(c) - \alpha a.$$

This is hardly unique, since, for example, if saturation is unimportant, the first $F^+(a)$ could be replaced by a^n.

Homework Assignment 8

(1) The basic process of competitive inhibition of P production by enzyme E from a fixed source S can be described by

$$S + E \underset{k'}{\overset{k}{\rightleftarrows}} C \overset{\ell}{\rightarrow} E + P,$$

$$I + E \underset{k'''}{\overset{k''}{\rightleftarrows}} C_I.$$

Analyze this from the viewpoint of discrete amplitude and time.

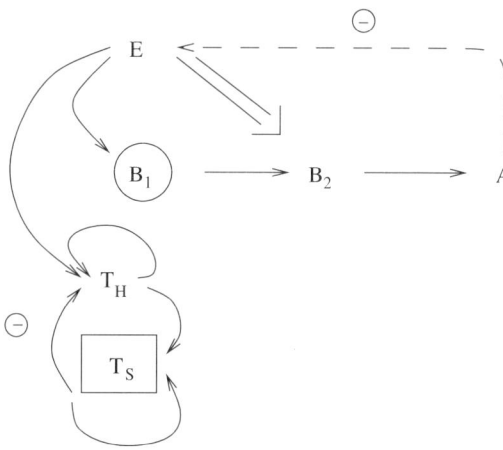

FIGURE 4.20. Model humoral response.

Finally, let us go to a model humoral response, in which the influence, and mutual influence, of T_H, helper, and T_S, suppressor, T-cells is taken into account (but the lymphokines, or molecular messengers, not indicated explicitly). The purported observations that are to be incorporated are the following:

(1) There is a negative feedback loop between T_H and T_S.
(2) T_H and T_S have autocatalytic feedback loops.
(3) Virgin (unactivated) B-cells are sensitive to negative signaling.

Also, one wants to predict multiple steady states: virgin, memory, and nonresponsive, as well as the kinetics of primary and secondary response, and the reaction phenomena of high Ag dose and low Ag dose paralysis. For the latter, one needs a primitive graded structure for the Ag, which we impose by attaching two Boolean variables to the Ag population: $e_1 = 0$ for no dose, $e_1 = 1, e_2 = 0$ for low dose, and $e_2 = 1$ for high dose.

The species in this model (Figure 4.20) are then E: antigen (e_1, e_2); B_1: virgin B-cells (b_1); B_2: mature activated B-cells (b_2); T_H: helper T-cells (h); T_S: suppressor T-cells (s); A: antibody (a). The suggested form is shown schematically in Figure 4.20, with $\Rightarrow$ indicating the necessity of e_2 for stimulation, $-\rightarrow$ for the mopping up of Ag by Ab, which we will not now include, preferring to control the Ag population by hand, (B_1) to indicate slow B_1 disappearance, and $\boxed{T_S}$ to indicate slow T_S growth. The corresponding symbolic dynamics equivalent to Figure 4.21 ($ab = 1$ only if $a = 1$ and $b = 1$, $a + b = 1$ if $a = 1$ and/or $b = 1$) is the very concise

(4.109)
$$b_1' = \bar{e}_1, \quad b_2' = b_1 e_2 h,$$
$$h' = e_1 \bar{s} + h, \quad s' = h + s, \quad a' = b_2 e_1 h.$$

With five control variables (at specified e_1, e_2), there are 32 possible states, making things a bit involved. Let us just indicate sample transitions for the three antigen levels $\bar{e}_1$, $e_1 \bar{e}_2$, and e_2:

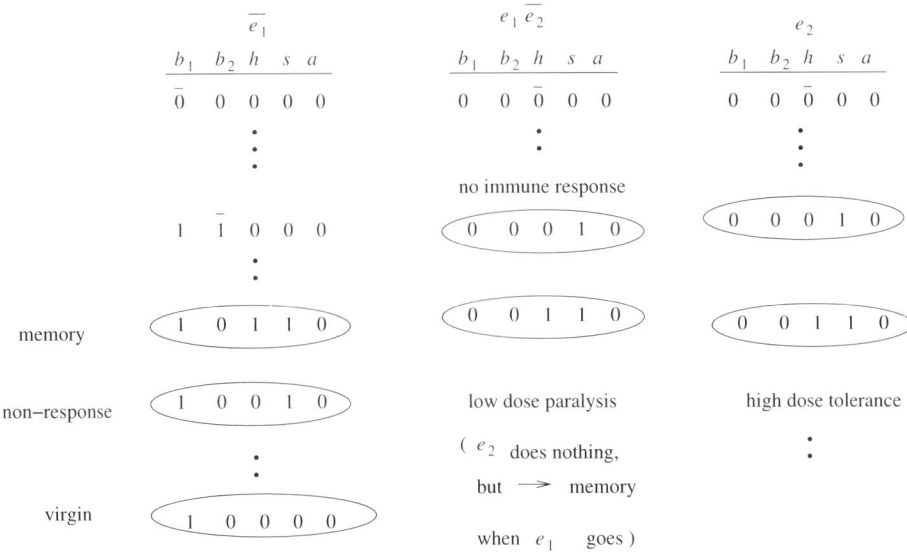

FIGURE 4.21. Discrete transitions of model humoral response.

A typical immune reaction sequence for slow b_1 disappearance and s growth would be

$$1\,0\,0\,0\,0 \xrightarrow{e_2} \overline{1}\,0\,\overline{0}\,0\,0 \to \overline{1}\,\overline{0}\,1\,\overline{0}\,0 \to \overline{1}\,1\,1\,0\,0 \to \overline{1}\,1\,1\,1\,\overline{0} \to \overline{1}\,1\,1\,1\,1.$$

In fact, this model, with timed reaction rates, satisfies quite well the initial desiderata. Completing the discrete-continuum transcription, now including e removal by a,

$$\dot{b}_1 = k_1 F_1^-(e) - d_1 b_1, \quad \dot{b}_2 = k_2 b_1 F_2^+(e)h - d_2 b_2,$$
$$\dot{h} = k_3 F_3^+(e) F_3 F_3^-(s) + m_3 F_3^+(h) - d_3 h,$$
(4.110)
$$\dot{s} = k_4 h + m_4 F_4^+(s) - d_4 s,$$
$$\dot{a} = k_5 b_2 eh - k_6 qa^q e^b - d_5 a, \quad \dot{i} = -k_5 pa^q e^b - d_6 e,$$

where several $F^+(x) \to x^n$ replacements have been incorporated.

References for Chapter 4

Glass, L., and Kauffmann, S. A. Co-operative components, spatial localization and oscillatory cellular dynamics. *J. Theor. Bio.* 34(2): 219–237, 1973. doi:10.1016/0022-5193(72)90157-9

Kaufman, M., Urbain, J., and Thomas, R. Towards a logical analysis of the immune response. *J. Theor. Bio.* 114(2): 527–561, 1985. doi:10.1016/S0022-5193(85)80042-4

Perelson, A. S., Mirmirani, M., and Oster, G. F. Optimal strategies in immunology. I. B-cell differentiation and proliferation. *J. Math. Biol.* 3(3-4): 325–367, 1976.

CHAPTER 5

Modeling Cell-Mediated Response

5.1. Cell-Mediated Toxicity

To respond to virally infected cells, the T-cell component gets directly into action—the cell, in the end, is recognized and killed by cytotoxic T-cells (CT lymphocytes), and by NKs and macrophages too. See Figure 5.1.
In outline, five stages are discernible:

(i) CTL finds target cell, by random or directed motion.
(ii) CTL recognizes and binds to target.
(iii) CTL delivers lethal hit.
(iv) Target disintegrates, with CTL staying or not staying bound.
(v) CTL recycles, staying or not staying bound.

We will first focus on the "queuing" phase of the process, (iii), during which the cells binding to the CTL are "served" death during their stay.

We now have a complex LT^n—lymphocyte $+ n$ targets—that has been formed, and ask for the probability $P_{nm}(t)$ that m of the attached cells have been lethally hit by time t (information experimentally available, since the process can be stopped by removing Ca^{++} with EDTA or by cooling). For this purpose, we must specify the service rate, with $\lambda_{nm}(t)dt$ as the probability that $m + 1$ cells have been hit by time $t + dt$ if m were hit by t. Since an m-hit state can appear from an $(m-1)$-hit

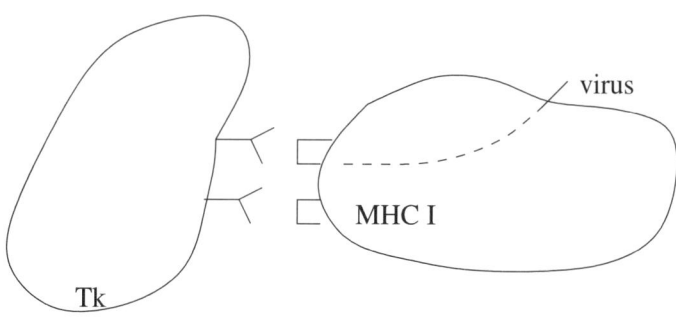

FIGURE 5.1. Virally infected cell meets CTL.

73

state or disappear into an $(m + 1)$-hit state, we have the following *master equation*:

$$\frac{dP_{n_0}(t)}{dt} = -\lambda_{n_0}(t)P_{n_0}(t),$$

(5.1) $$\frac{dP_{nm}(t)}{dt} = -\lambda_{nm}(t)P_{nm}(t) + \lambda_{n,m-1}(t)P_{n,m-1}(t), \quad 1 \le m \le n - 1,$$

$$\frac{dP_{nn}(t)}{dt} = \lambda_{n,n-1}P_{n,n-1}(t), \quad 1 \le m \le m, \; P_{n0}(0) = 1, \; P_{nm}(0) = 0.$$

For a more compact formulation, imagine an infinite number of "ghost" target configurations: $n + 1$, $n + 2$, $\ldots$, and lump them together with the real targets in computing P_{nn}. In other words, we define $\bar{P}_{nn}(t) = 0$ for $m < 0$, $\bar{P}_{nm}(t) = P_{nm}(t)$ for $0 \le m < n$, and $P_{nn}(t) = \sum_{m=n}^{\infty} \bar{P}_{nm}(t)$; we now have simply

(5.2) $$\frac{d\bar{P}_{nm}(t)}{dt} = -\lambda_{nm}(t)\bar{P}_{nm}(t) + \lambda_{nm-1}(t)P_{n,m-1}(t),$$

$$\forall m, \; \bar{P}_{nm}(0) = \delta_{m,0}.$$

Two basic models will be considered.

(a) $\lambda_{nm}(t) = \lambda$ (a constant that could depend on n): In dt, the CTL shifts its machinery to an unhit cell and works on it. So now

(5.3) $$\frac{d\bar{P}_{nm}(t)}{dt} = -\lambda\bar{P}_{nm}(t) + \lambda\bar{P}_{nm-1}(t),$$

$$\bar{P}_{nm}(0) = \delta_{m,0}.$$

To solve this set, introduce the generating function

(5.4) $$\bar{P}_n(x,t) = \sum_{-\infty}^{\infty} \bar{P}_{nm}(t)x^m.$$

Multiplying (4.3) by x^m and adding, we thus have

(5.5) $$\frac{d\bar{P}_n(x,t)}{dt} = -\lambda\bar{P}_n(x,t) + \lambda x\bar{P}_n(x,t), \quad \bar{P}_n(x,0) = 1,$$

solved immediately as

(5.6) $$\bar{P}_n(x,t) = e^{\lambda(x-1)t}.$$

Hence, taking the coefficient of x^m,

(5.7) $$\bar{P}_{nm}(t) = (\lambda t)^m \frac{e^{-\lambda t}}{m!},$$

the familiar Poisson, which therefore implies

(5.8) $$P_{nm}(t) = (\lambda t)^m \frac{e^{-\lambda t}}{m!}, \quad m < n,$$

$$P_{nn}(t) = \sum_{n}^{\infty} (\lambda t)^m \frac{e^{-\lambda t}}{m!} = 1 - \sum_{0}^{n-1} (\lambda t)^m \frac{e^{-\lambda t}}{m!}.$$

(b) In this model, in dt, the CTL works on one target cell, but it may be one that is already lethally hit; only a fraction $\frac{n-m}{n}$ of these hits are effective, so that here $\lambda_{nm}(t) = \lambda(1 - \frac{m}{n})$. We thus have, dropping the implicit n,

$$\text{(5.9)} \qquad \frac{dP_m(t)}{dt} = -\frac{\lambda}{m}(n - m)P_m(t) + \frac{\lambda}{m}(n + 1 - m)P_{m-1}(t),$$
$$P_m(0) = \delta_{m,0}.$$

It is convenient to set $Q_m(t) = P_{n-m}(t)$, so instead

$$\text{(5.10)} \qquad \frac{dQ_m(t)}{dt} = -\frac{\lambda}{n}mQ_m(t) + \frac{\lambda}{m}(m + 1)Q_{m+1}(t),$$
$$Q_m(0) = \delta_{m,n}.$$

Introducing $Q(x,t) = \sum x^m Q_m(t)$, we also need $\frac{\partial Q(x,t)}{\partial x} = \sum m x^{m-1} Q_m(t)$. Summing (4.10) with weight x^m, we then have

$$\text{(5.11)} \qquad \frac{\partial Q(x,t)}{\partial t} = -\frac{\lambda}{n}(x - 1)\frac{\partial Q(x,t)}{\partial x},$$
$$Q(x,0) = x^n.$$

Equation (5.11) is equally routine; we observe that

$$\text{(5.12)} \qquad \left.\frac{\partial t}{\partial x}\right|_Q = -\frac{\partial Q/\partial x|_t}{\partial Q/\partial t|_x} = \frac{n}{\lambda}\frac{1}{x - 1}$$

so

$$\text{(5.13)} \qquad t = C(Q) + \frac{n}{\lambda}\ln(x - 1).$$

Inserting the boundary condition $0 = C(Q) + \frac{n}{\lambda}\ln(Q^{1/n} - 1)$ and solving for Q, we get

$$\text{(5.14)} \qquad Q = (1 - e^{-\lambda t/n} + xe^{-\lambda t/n})^n,$$

from which

$$\text{(5.15)} \qquad \begin{aligned} P_{nm}(t) &= Q_{n-m}(t) \\ &= \binom{n}{m}(1 - e^{-\lambda t/n})^m (e^{-\lambda t/n})^{n-m}, \end{aligned}$$

just a binomial distribution with "success" probability $p(t) = 1 - e^{-\lambda t/m}$, that of a specified target cell not surviving until time t. Now the most reliable information is on the mean value $\bar{m}(t) = \sum m P_{nm}(t)$. This is, respectively, for models (a) and (b),

$$\text{(5.16a)} \qquad m(t) = n - e^{-\lambda t}\sum_{m=0}^{n-1}(n - m)\frac{(\lambda t)^m}{m!},$$

$$\text{(5.16b)} \qquad m(t) = n(1 - e^{-\lambda t/n}).$$

Measurements in fact definitely favor (a); the CTL does not waste its ammunition on a moribund target.

From a longer-time viewpoint, two important aspects have been glossed over: the probability of cells attaching in the first place, and of their detachment. We consider this from a killer-cell-population perspective. Consider a unit volume, with $n_i(t)$ the number of CTLs—and hence the concentration—with i target cells attached. For M possible binding sites, we then have the sequence

$$\cdots \left(n_{i-1} \right) \underset{\mu_i}{\overset{\lambda_{i-1}}{\rightleftarrows}} \left(n_i \right) \underset{\mu_{i+1}}{\overset{\lambda_i}{\rightleftarrows}} \left(n_{i+1} \right) \cdots$$

or

$$\frac{dn_0}{dt} = -\lambda_0 n_0 + \mu_1 n_1,$$

(5.17)
$$\frac{dn_i}{dt} = \lambda_{i-1} n_{i-1} - (\lambda_i + \mu_i) n_i + \mu_{i+l} n_{i+1}, \quad 0 < i < M,$$

$$\frac{dn_M}{dt} = \lambda_{n-1} n_{M-1} - \mu_M n_m, \quad n_i(0) = n\delta_{i0}.$$

Setting $\mu_0 = 0$, $\lambda_n = 0$, and $n_{-1} = n_{M+1} = 0$ forever, these collapse into the single expression

(5.18)
$$\frac{dn_i}{dt} = \lambda_{i-1} n_{i-1} - (\lambda_i + \mu_i) n_i + \mu_{i+1} n_{i+1}.$$

If x_0 is the total number of target cells available, then of course the number of free target cells will be

(5.19)
$$x(t) = x_0 - \sum_0^M i n_i(t), \quad x(0) = x_0.$$

It is reasonable to choose $\lambda_i = k(M - i)x(t)$ proportional to the number of free sites, and $\mu_i(t) = k'i$ proportional to the number of absorbed targets. The dynamics is then highly nonlinear in the $n_i(t)$, but if we can determine the "collective variable" $x(t)$ separately, it will become linear again.

To find $x(t)$, we use the relations $\sum_i n_i = n$, given, and $\sum i n_i = x_0 - x(t)$ to write

$$\frac{dx}{dt} = -\sum i \frac{dn_i}{dt}$$

$$= \sum (-i\lambda_{i-1} n_{i-1} + i(\lambda_i + \mu_i) n_i - i\mu_{i+1} n_{i+1})$$

$$= \sum (-(i + 1)\lambda_i + i(\lambda_i + \mu_i) - (i - 1)\mu_i) n_i$$

$$= \sum (-\lambda_i + \mu_i) n_i,$$

$$= \sum (-k(M - i)x + k'i) n_i$$

$$= -kxM \sum n_i + kx \sum i n_i + k' \sum i n_i$$

or, quite simply,

$$(5.20) \qquad \frac{dx}{dt} = k'x_0 + (k(x_0 - Mn) - k')x - kx^2, \quad x(0) = x_0.$$

It is convenient to rescale: $X(t) = x(t)/x_0$, $\alpha = nM/x_0$, $p_i(t) = n_i(t)/n$, $\tau = kx_0 t$, and $\kappa = k'/kx_0$, so the complete set of relations becomes

$$\frac{dp_i}{d\tau} = (M - i + 1)Xp_{i-1}$$
$$(5.21) \qquad \qquad - ((M - i)X + \kappa i)p_i + \kappa(i + 1)p_{i+1}, \quad p_i(0) = \delta_{i,0},$$
$$\frac{dX}{d\tau} = \kappa - (\alpha + \kappa - 1)X - X^2, \quad X(0) = 1.$$

The X-equation is trivial to solve, in the form

$$(5.22) \quad \frac{dX}{d\tau} = -(X - \gamma_1)(X - \gamma_2)$$

$$\text{where } \gamma_{1,2} = \frac{1}{2}[-(\alpha + \kappa - 1) \pm [(\alpha + \kappa - 1)^2 + 4\kappa]^{1/2}],$$

leading to

$$(5.23) \qquad X(\tau) = \frac{\gamma_1(1 - \gamma_2) - \gamma_2(1 - \gamma_1)e^{-(\gamma_1 - \gamma_2)\tau}}{1 - \gamma_2 - (1 - \gamma_1)e^{-(\gamma_1 - \gamma_2)\tau}}.$$

However, then the p_i equations (4.24) are again solved by the generating function method, obtaining

$$(5.24) \qquad p_i(\tau) = \binom{M}{i} \left(\frac{1 - X(\tau)}{\alpha}\right)^i \left(1 - \frac{1 - X(\tau)}{\alpha}\right)^{M-i},$$

which is consistent with the elementary probability

$$P(\tau) = \frac{1 - X(\tau)}{\alpha} = \frac{x_0 - x(\tau)}{nM}$$

that a particular site is occupied at time τ.

Dynamically, of course, p_0 "leaks" to p_1, which leaks to p_2, etc., with successive peaking before falling to equilibrium. A useful concept is the mean coverage, the proportion of binding sites that are occupied: $\theta(\tau) = \bar{i}/M = \sum i p_i(\tau)/M = (1 - X(\tau))/\alpha$, just the probability that a given site is occupied. In particular, θ_∞ is obtained from $X_\infty = \gamma_1 = \frac{1}{2}([(\alpha + \kappa - 1)^2 + 4\kappa]^{1/2} - (\alpha + \kappa - 1))$. This is to be compared with the irreversible adsorption case $\kappa = 0$, in which $X_\infty = 0$ and $\theta_\infty = .5$. Experimentally, using $M = 4$, $\alpha = 2$, and $p_0(\infty) = (1 - \theta(\infty))^M = .66$, one sees that instead $\theta_\infty = .1$, corresponding to the quite high detachment value $\kappa = 7.2$.

Homework Assignment 9

(1) The Poisson and binomial forms (5.7), (5.15), (5.24) are ubiquitous. What hierarchies of reactions do they satisfy?

5.2. Immune Surveillance

Population Viewpoint. We now consider very much of a toy model of CTL control of an emerging pathogenic cell population. Here "microcancers" X are imagined to arise that are recognized by the cytotoxic population M, of which M_1 bind to X, and M_0 remain unbound. X is regarded as produced both by transformation (e.g., via damage to checkpoint controls) of normal cells, $0 \to X$, and by induced transformation, $0 + X \to 2X$. The unbound population is taken as homeostatically fixed: $0 + X = N$, a constant, and M_0 is recovered from M_1 by detachment of dead X's. Thus, we have

$$0 \xrightarrow{A} X,$$

(5.25)
$$0 + X \xrightarrow{\lambda} 2X,$$

$$X + M_0 \xrightarrow{k_1} M_1 \to M_0 + P.$$

We also allow diffusion of the mobile cytotoxic cells, which is however inhibited by a factor $1 + KX$ (e.g., by lymphokines) in the presence of target cells X. Hence

$$\dot{X} = (N - X)(A + \lambda X) - k_1 M_0 X,$$

(5.26)
$$\dot{M}_0 = -k_1 M_0 X + k_2 M_1 + \mu' \nabla^2 \left(\frac{M_0}{1 + KX} \right),$$

$$\dot{M}_1 = k_1 M_0 X - k_2 M_1 + \mu' \nabla^2 \left(\frac{M_1}{1 + KX} \right).$$

If the second and third reactions are taken as very fast, they can be taken in equilibrium, $\dot{M}_0 = \dot{M}_1 \to 0$, and the second and third equations then imply $\nabla^2(M_0 + M_1/(1 + KX)) = 0$. Hence, with any reasonable boundary conditions, $M_0 + M_1 = M(1 + KX)$ for some spatial constant M, so $M_1 = (1 + KX)M - M_0$, and the system is reduced to

$$\dot{X} = (N - X)(A + \lambda X) - k_1 M_0 X,$$

(5.27)
$$(k_2 + k_1 X)M_0 = \mu' \nabla^2 \frac{M_0}{1 + KX} + k_2 M(1 + KX).$$

Even (5.27) is a bit involved, and so we further reduce it by going over to a two-compartment model of diffusion—an active volume ΔV inside a larger sluggish volume $\bar{V} = V - \Delta V$, both connected by a primitive unimolecular reaction version of diffusion. The quantities inside $\bar{V}$ can be regarded as fixed, and so (5.27) is replaced by

(5.28)
$$\dot{X} = (N - X)(A + \lambda X) - k_1 M_0 X$$

where

$$(k_1 + k_2)M_0 = \mu \left(\frac{\bar{M}_0}{1 + K\bar{X}} - \frac{M_0}{1 + KX} \right) + k_2 M(1 + KX)$$

$$\text{and} \quad (k_1 + k_2 \bar{X})\bar{M}_0 = k_2 M(1 + k\bar{X});$$

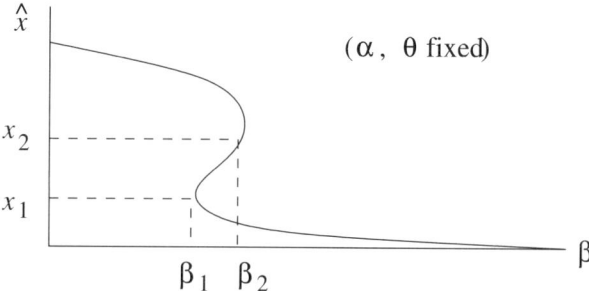

FIGURE 5.2. Steady-state relationship.

here quantities in $\overline{V}$ are indicated by upper bars. On eliminating M_0 and $\overline{M}_0$, we end up with

$$(5.29) \qquad \frac{dx}{d\tau} = \alpha + (1 - \theta x)x - \beta x \frac{(1 + \gamma x)[(1 + \overline{x})(1 + \gamma \overline{x}) + D]}{(1 + \gamma \overline{x})(1 + \overline{x})[(1 + x)(1 + \gamma x) + D]}$$

where

$$L = \frac{k_1}{k_2}, \quad \gamma = \frac{K}{L}, \quad D = \frac{\mu}{k_2}, \quad x = LX,$$

$$\tau = (\lambda N - A)t, \quad \alpha = \frac{ANL}{\lambda N - A}, \quad \theta = \frac{\lambda / L}{\lambda N - A},$$

are measures of the normal cell population, $\beta = \frac{k_1 M}{\lambda N - A}$ of the bathing lymphocyte population, and of course X of the malignant cells.

The qualitative nature of (5.29) is not altered in the diffusionless $\mu = D = 0$ case, and so we shall reduce to this case:

$$(5.30) \qquad x' = \alpha + (1 - \theta x)x - \frac{\beta x}{1 + x}.$$

In particular, the all-important steady-state solution, which satisfies

$$(5.31) \qquad \beta = [\alpha + (1 - \theta \widehat{x})\widehat{x}]\frac{1 + \widehat{x}}{\widehat{x}},$$

has the form shown in Figure 5.2. Clearly, $\widehat{x}$ is high for $\beta < \beta_1$, low for $\beta > \beta_2$, but multivalued between limits satisfying $d\beta/d\widehat{x} = 0$ or

$$(5.32) \qquad 2\theta \widehat{x}^3 - (1 - \theta)\widehat{x}^2 + \alpha = 0.$$

In practice, $\alpha \ll 1$, and the low-$\widehat{x}$ and high-$\widehat{x}$ solutions are given, Figure 5.3, by

$$(5.33) \qquad x_1 = \sqrt{\frac{\alpha}{1 - \theta}}, \quad x_2 = \frac{1 - \theta}{2\theta},$$

$$\text{with} \quad \beta_1 = 1 + \sqrt{\alpha(1 - \theta)}, \quad \beta_2 = \frac{(1 + \theta)^2}{4\theta}.$$

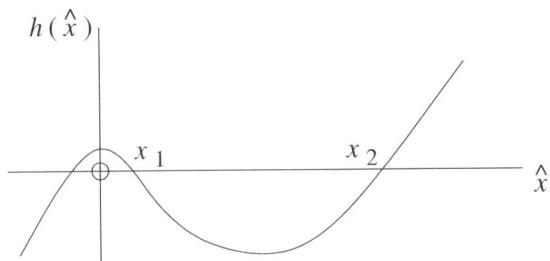

FIGURE 5.3. Coefficient of stability.

But what happens in the parameter region $\beta_1 < \beta < \beta_2$? To find out, we use the dynamics of $\xi = x - \hat{x}$ for x near $\hat{x}$. From (5.30), we have, to linear order in ξ,

$$(5.34) \qquad \xi' = -\frac{h(\hat{x})}{\hat{x}(1 + \hat{x})}\xi \quad \text{where } h(\hat{x}) = 2\theta\hat{x}^3 - (1 - \theta)\hat{x}^2 + \alpha.$$

Clearly, $\xi = 0$ is stable ($h > 0$) for $\hat{x} > x_2$, or $\hat{x} < x_1$, but unstable in the middle region $x_1 < \hat{x} < x_2$, which will therefore not be attained asymptotically. Whether the cancerous upper branch or the controlled lower branch is realized in the region $\beta_1 < \beta < \beta_2$ must therefore be sensitive to initial conditions or to fluctuations during the dynamics.

5.3. Effect of Fluctuations

When small numbers of objects are involved, fluctuations in measured quantities are the norm. The chemical kinetics or population framework that we have focused on is one in which such fluctuations are eliminated from consideration, typically by replacing averages of functions by functions of averages. There are clearly situations—chance extinction of a species, or chance initiation of a species—in which fluctuations play a crucial role, and in (4.88)–(4.89), a small attempt was made to take these into account. The correct approach, in principle, involves inserting much more detail into both description and basic mechanism. There is, however, a quite successful format, stochastic kinetics, in which the former is accomplished with minimal attention to the latter. It is a master equation format, already used in (5.1) and (5.17), based upon reinterpreting a reaction

$$A \xrightarrow{k} B$$

in which A A-molecules transmute to B-molecules at a rate of kA per unit time, to a picture in which a single A-molecule has a probability k per unit time to convert to a B. Thus, we must work not with a strictly deterministic system, but with a probability distribution $P(A, B, t)$ for A A-molecules and B B-molecules to be present at time t.

In this case, a unit reaction produces the state (A, B) if one previously had $(A + 1, B - 1)$ and destroys (A, B) by converting it to $(A - 1, B + 1)$. It is clear on counting the number of ways a conversion can occur that

$$(5.35) \qquad \frac{\partial}{\partial t} P(A, B, t) = k(A + 1)P(A + 1, B - 1, t) - kAP(A, B, t).$$

Similarly, a more complicated reaction, for example, $2A + B \xrightarrow{k} A + C$, would translate into

$$(5.36) \quad \frac{\partial}{\partial t} P(A, B, C, t) =$$
$$k(A + 1)^2(B + 1)P(A + 1, B + 1, C - 1, t) - kA^2 P(A, B, C, t),$$

and a set of reactions would contribute additively to $\partial P/\partial t$.

Now we can return to our original equations (5.25) in the absence of diffusion,

$$O \rightarrow X,$$
$$(5.26) \qquad O + X \rightarrow 2X,$$
$$X + M_0 \rightarrow M_1, \quad M_1 \rightarrow M_0 + P.$$

Species O is again to be eliminated by assuming that $O + X = N$ is fixed, and so, from (5.35) and (5.36), we clearly have

$$
\begin{aligned}
(5.37) \quad \frac{\partial}{\partial t} P(XM_0M_1t) &= (N + 1 - X)(A + \lambda(X - 1))P(X - 1M_0M_1t) \\
&\quad - (N - X)(A + \lambda X)P(XM_0M_1t) \\
&\quad + k_1(X + 1)(M_0 + 1)P(X + 1M_0 + 1M_1 - 1t) \\
&\quad - k_1 XM_0 P(XM_0M_1t) \\
&\quad + k_2(M_1 + 1)P(XM_0 - 1M_1 + 1t) \\
&\quad - k_2 M_1 P(XM_0M_1t).
\end{aligned}
$$

If we sum over M_0 and M_1, setting $\sum_{M_0M_1} P(XM_0M_1t) = P(Xt)$, while $\sum_{M_0M_1} M_0 P(XM_0M_1t) \equiv \langle M_0 \rangle_x P(X_1t)$, (5.37) is reduced to

$$
\begin{aligned}
(5.38) \quad \frac{\partial}{\partial t} P(Xt) &= (N + 1 - X)(A + \lambda(X - 1))P(X - 1, t) \\
&\quad - (N - X)(A + \lambda X)P(Xt) \\
&\quad + k_1(X + 1)\langle M_0 \rangle_{X+1} P(X + 1, t) - k_1 X \langle M_0 \rangle_X P(X, t) \\
&\quad + k_2 \langle M_1 \rangle_X P(Xt) - k_2 \langle M_1 \rangle_X P(xt).
\end{aligned}
$$

But repeating the quasi-state assumption for the last two reactions, we have $M_0 + M_1 = M$, and then $M_0 = k_2 M/(k_2 + k_1 X)$, so that

$$
\begin{aligned}
(5.39) \quad \frac{\partial}{\partial t} P(X, t) &= (N + 1 - X)(A + \lambda(X - 1)P(X - 1, t) \\
&\quad - (N - X)(A + \lambda X)P(Xt) \\
&\quad - M \frac{k_1 k_2 X}{k_2 + k_1 X} P(Xt) + M \frac{k_1 k_2(X + 1)}{k_2 + k_1(X + 1)} P(X + 1t).
\end{aligned}
$$

Let us return to equilibrium, $\dot{P} = 0$, in the form

$$(5.40) \quad (N + 1 - X)(A + \lambda(X - 1))P(X - 1, t) - M \frac{k_1 k_2 X}{k_2 + k_1 X} P(X, t) =$$
$$(N - X)(A + \lambda X)P(X, t) - M \frac{k_1 k_2 (X + 1)}{k_2 + k_1 (X + 1)} P(X + 1, t),$$

i.e., $F(X) = F(X + 1)$, which must thereby be a constant, and by setting $X = 0$ on the left-hand side, the constant must be 0. We conclude that, in equilibrium,

$$(5.41) \qquad P(X + 1) = \frac{(N - X)(A + \lambda X)(k_2 + k_1(X + 1))}{k_1 k_2 M(X + 1)} P(X),$$

or, going over to our previous scaled notation,

$$(5.42) \qquad \frac{P(x + L)}{P(x)} = \frac{(\alpha + x(1 - \theta x))(1 + x + L)}{\beta(x + L)}.$$

If $X \gg 1$, so that $x \gg L$, we can expand $P(X + L)$ to first order in L, and write

$$(5.43) \qquad \frac{d}{dx} \ln P(x) = \frac{\alpha + (1 + \alpha - \beta)x + (1 - \theta)x^2 - \theta x^3}{\beta L x}.$$

It is then simple to show that if $x < x_1$, $P(x)$ has a single maximum at $\bar{x}_1(\beta)$, the lower root, and if $x > x_2$, at $\bar{x}_2(\beta)$, the upper root. But if $x_1 < x < x_2$, there is a maximum at $\bar{x}_1(\beta)$, a minimum at the intermediate root, and for $\alpha \ll 1$ a much larger maximum at $\bar{x}_2(\beta)$. In other words, fluctuations drive the system predominantly into the large cancer population regime. Actually, if diffusion is reintroduced, there is another steady state solution of microcancer form.

5.4. Tumor Escape

Now we proceed to very much of a population problem (Figure 5.4), the deterministic dynamics of a solid tumor in the presence of a reactive lymphocyte population stimulated by, and antagonistic to, the tumor—a minimal mathematical model. Assume that only the surface of the tumor is accessible (neglecting effector penetration via vascularization). Let L be the free (unbound) lymphocytes, and $\bar{C}$ the number of free tumor cells at the tumor surface. Assume as well first-order lymphocyte attrition, but stimulation proportional to the exposed tumor cell population, together with a standard logistic saturation factor for lymphocyte production:

$$(5.44) \qquad \frac{dL}{dt} = -\lambda_1 L + \alpha_1' \bar{C} L \left(1 - \frac{L}{L_0}\right).$$

Furthermore, C, the total number of tumor cells, will increase by proliferation of the total free cells C_f, but decrease by binding of those not already bound:

$$(5.45) \qquad \frac{dC}{dt} = \lambda_2 C_f - \alpha_2' \bar{C} L.$$

The binding of the surface tumor cell population, say C_s, to the lymphocyte population L is imagined as equilibrium controlled in the usual way by

$$\bar{C} + L \rightleftarrows (\bar{C} L)$$

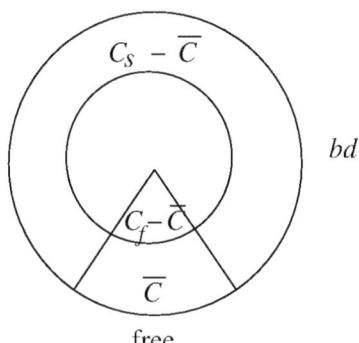

FIGURE 5.4. Model for tumor dynamics.

or

(5.46) $$(\bar{C}L) = K\bar{C}L.$$

But $\bar{C} + (\bar{C}L) = C$, so

(5.47) $$\bar{C} = \frac{C_s}{1 + KL}.$$

Now for a roughly spherical shape, we can write $C_s = \gamma C^{2\beta}$. Since $C_f = C - (\bar{C}L)$ as well, we can eliminate $\bar{C}$, C_s, and C_f from our equations to arrive at

(5.48)
$$\frac{dL}{dt} = -\lambda_1 L + \frac{\alpha_1' C^{2/3} L}{1 + KL}\left(1 - \frac{L}{L_0}\right),$$
$$\frac{dC}{dt} = \lambda_2 C - \frac{\gamma C^{2/3} L}{1 + KL}(\lambda_2 K + \alpha_2').$$

Homework Assignment 10

(1) The statement that (5.21), with $X(\tau)$, can be solved by the generating function method is a bit glib. When will (5.24) solve (5.21)? What can one do when it doesn't?

(2) Verify the statements following (5.43).

With the scaling $x = KL$, $x_0 = L_0 K$, $y = KC$, $\alpha_1 = \alpha_1' \gamma' K^{2/3}$, and $\alpha_2 = \gamma K^{1/3}(\lambda_2 + \alpha_2'/K)$, we then have

(5.49)
$$\frac{dx}{dt} = -\lambda_1 x + \frac{\alpha_1 x y^{2/3}}{1 + x}\left(1 - \frac{x}{x_0}\right) + [\lambda_1 x_0],$$
$$\frac{dy}{dt} = \lambda_2 y - \frac{\alpha_2 x y^{2/3}}{1 + x};$$

here the bracketed addition allows for the possibility of a steady lymphocyte source, a not unreasonable assumption.

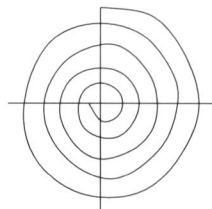

FIGURE 5.5. Nodal singularity.

In our setup, x represents the lymphocyte population available to control the tumor size y. What is the repertoire? We will neglect the source term $\lambda_1 x_0$ and write

(5.50)
$$\dot{x} = xf(x,y), \qquad f(x,y) = -\lambda_1 + \alpha_1 y^{2/3} \frac{1 - x/x_0}{1+x},$$
$$\dot{y} = y^{2/3} g(x,y), \qquad g(x,y) = \lambda_2 y^{1/3} - \alpha_2 \frac{x}{1+x},$$

putting into evidence the fact that initial $x > 0$, $y > 0$ will be maintained. The qualitative nature of this pair of ODEs of course is determined by the nature of the singular points $f(\bar{x}, \bar{y}) = 0 = g(\bar{x}\bar{y})$, as well as the "universal" singular point $\bar{x} = \bar{y} = 0$. The latter is necessarily a saddle point, i.e.,

(5.51)
$$\left(\begin{matrix} \frac{\partial \dot{x}}{\partial x} & \frac{\partial \dot{x}}{\partial y^{2/3}} \\ \frac{\partial \dot{y}^{2/3}}{\partial x} & \frac{\partial \dot{y}^{2/3}}{\partial \dot{y}^{2/3}} \end{matrix} \right)_{x=y=0} = \left(\begin{matrix} -\lambda_1 & 0 \\ -\frac{2}{3}\alpha_2 & \frac{1}{3}\lambda_2 \end{matrix} \right)$$

so that trajectories flow in along the x-axis and out along the y-axis.

For the remainder of the dynamics, let us first recall that for a pair of ODEs $\dot{x} = F$, $\dot{y} = G$, expansion about a singular point $(\bar{x}, \bar{y})$ yields

(5.52)
$$\begin{pmatrix} \delta \dot{x} \\ \delta \dot{y} \end{pmatrix} = \begin{pmatrix} F_{\bar{x}} & F_{\bar{y}} \\ G_{\bar{x}} & G_{\bar{y}} \end{pmatrix} \begin{pmatrix} \delta x \\ \delta y \end{pmatrix}$$

with solution

$$\begin{pmatrix} \delta x \\ \delta y \end{pmatrix} = u e^{\Lambda_1 t} + v e^{\Lambda_2 t}$$

determined by

(5.53)
$$\begin{pmatrix} F_{\bar{x}} & F_{\bar{y}} \\ G_{\bar{x}} & G_{\bar{y}} \end{pmatrix} u = \Lambda_1 u, \qquad \begin{pmatrix} F_{\bar{x}} & F_{\bar{y}} \\ G_{\bar{x}} & G_{\bar{y}} \end{pmatrix} v = \Lambda_2 v;$$

Λ_1 and Λ_2 are the eigenvalues of the Jacobian matrix at the singular point in question. The possibilities are then

(i) Λ_1 and Λ_2 complex conjugates.

If

$$\text{Re}(\Lambda) \begin{cases} < 0 \\ > 0, \end{cases}$$

this is a node (Figure 5.5), with

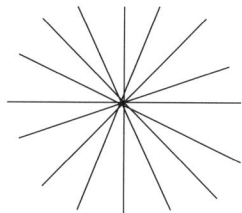

FIGURE 5.6. Focal singularity.

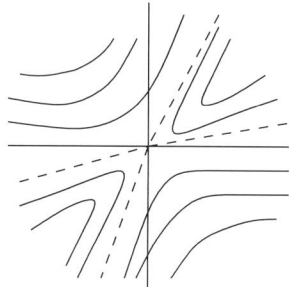

FIGURE 5.7. Saddle point.

$$\begin{cases} \text{stable sink} \\ \text{unstable source} \end{cases} \quad \text{and trajectories spiraling} \quad \begin{cases} \text{inward} \\ \text{outward.} \end{cases}$$

(ii) Λ_1 and Λ_2 real, $\Lambda_1 \Lambda_2 > 0$.

If

$$\text{both} \begin{cases} < 0 \\ > 0, \end{cases}$$

this is a focus (Figure 5.6), with

$$\begin{cases} \text{stable sink} \\ \text{unstable source} \end{cases} \quad \text{and trajectories radially} \quad \begin{cases} \text{inward} \\ \text{outward.} \end{cases}$$

(iii) $\Lambda_1 \Lambda_2 < 0$. A saddle (Figure 5.7 with two separatrices, separating four classes of in and out trajectories.

(iv) Limiting borderline cases: $\text{Re}(\Lambda = 0)$, $\Lambda_1 \Lambda_2 = 0$, only one Λ.

Now returning to (5.50) and eliminating $\bar{y}$ from $f(\bar{x}, \bar{y}) = g(\bar{x}, \bar{y}) = 0$, we find

(5.54) $$\phi(\bar{x}) \equiv \frac{\bar{x}^2 (1 - \bar{x}/x_0)}{(1 + \bar{x})^3} = \phi^* \quad \text{where } \phi^* = \frac{\lambda_1 \lambda_2^2}{\alpha_1 \alpha_2^2}.$$

Since

(5.55) $$\phi_{\max} = \left(\frac{4}{27}\right)\left(\frac{x_0}{1 + x_0}\right)^2,$$

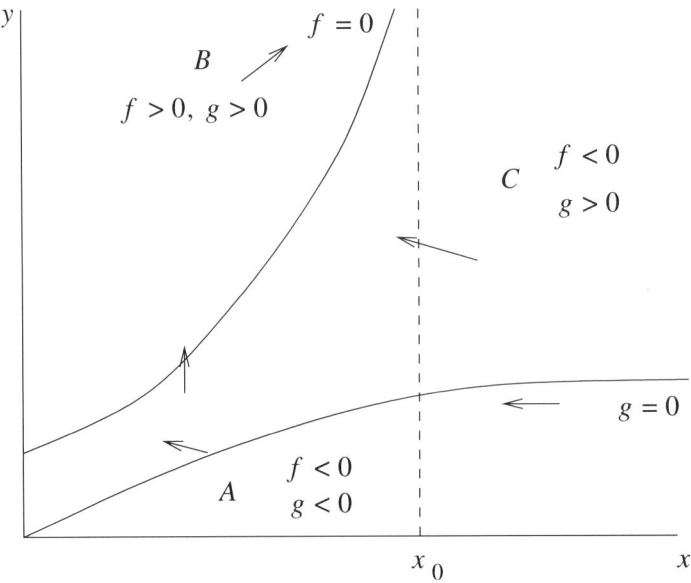

FIGURE 5.8. Case (a).

there are two regimes.

(a) $\phi^* = (\lambda_1 \lambda_2^2 / \alpha_1 \alpha_2^2) > \phi_{\max}$ (large λ_1 / α_1 or λ_2 / α_2).

In Figure 5.8 there is no internal singular point, only $\bar{x} = \bar{y} = 0$, and there are three regions of trajectories, with flow patterns as shown. At a gross level, the flow is undirectional, with the sequence $A \to C \to B \to (x_0, \infty)$: the tumor always escapes lymphocyte control.

(b) $\phi^* < \phi_{\max} < \frac{4}{27}$.

Then, (5.54), written as

$$(5.56) \qquad \left(1 + \frac{1}{\phi^* x_0}\right)\bar{x}^3 - \left(\frac{1}{\phi^*} - 3\right)\bar{x}^2 + 3\bar{x} + 1 = 0,$$

has two singular-point solutions. In Figure 5.9 there are five basic zones of trajectories:

$$A: \; f < 0, \; g < 0,$$
$$B: \; f > 0, \; g > 0,$$
$$C, D: \; f < 0, \; g > 0,$$
$$D: \; f > 0, \; g < 0.$$

The singular point s_2 is necessarily a saddle, with separatrices distinguishing the trajectories from A which enter either C (A_1 or A_2) or D (A_3), and those which enter A from E (A_2) or from $x > x_{00}$ (A_1 or A_3). These separatrices extend into B, picking out the trajectories from B which enter E (B_2) from those which

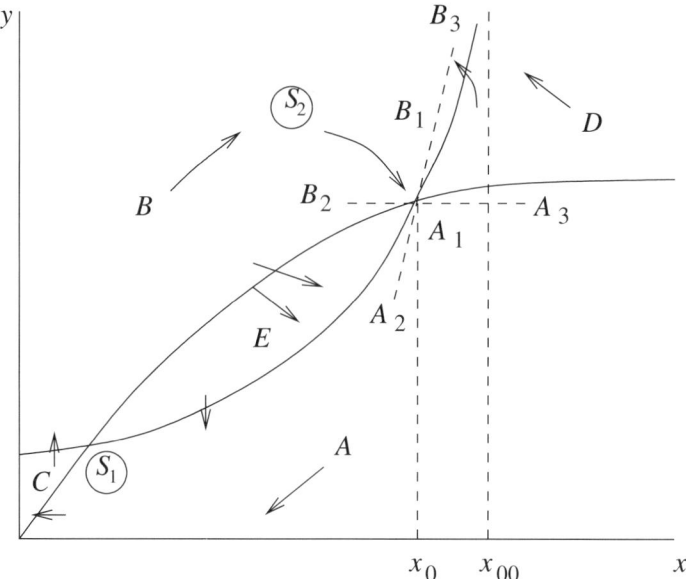

FIGURE 5.9. Case (b).

take off to (x_0, ∞). Thus, the transition schemes take the form

(5.57)
$$
\begin{array}{ccccc}
A_1 & \longrightarrow & C & \longrightarrow & B_1 \\
& \nearrow & & \searrow & \\
A_2 & \longleftarrow & E \longleftarrow B_2 & & (x_0, \infty) \\
& & & \nearrow & \\
A_3 & \longrightarrow & D & \longrightarrow & B_3
\end{array}
$$

and the possibility of a cycle $B_2 E A_2 C B_2$ that limits the tumor growth now appears.

Since this cycle encloses S_1, it is the properties of S_1 that are crucial. It is straightforward to show that S_1 is a stable node or focus if

(5.58)
$$
\lambda_1 \frac{\overline{x}}{1 + \overline{x}} \frac{1 + 1/x_0}{1 - \overline{x}/x_0} > \frac{\lambda_2}{3},
$$

or else unstable, leading to tumor escape. If one starts instead in A_1, which oddly enough can also be achieved by removing tumor cells (e.g., when x is approaching its minimum), or by adding lymphocytes at precisely the right time during the $C B_2 E A_2$ cycle, the tumor will escape.

Homework Assignment 11

(1) How far can you carry the analysis of (5.28) without the compartment approximation to diffusion?

(2) Diffusion is claimed to introduce a new steady state into the analysis of (5.42). Verify this.

CHAPTER 6

Control of Immune Response

6.1. Immune Networks

Model Analysis. The initial response of a resting B-cell population to antigen it encounters can proceed via any of the following: a sensitive class of memory cells that quickly produce copious Ab in response; unstimulated B-cells that proliferate on exposure; cells that recognize Ag but are tolerant—they do not proliferate and produce Ab explosively. Presumably, there are no other broad types; somatic mutation keeps on modifying the cells produced by the bone marrow, and in principle all Ag can be recognized. Jerne suggested in 1973 that the controlling elements are themselves controlled because they are recognized by other B-initiated components which keep down *their* concentrations. A characteristic portion of an Ab molecule that can be recognized is called an *idiotope*, and it is recognized by anti-idiotypic Ab's; less specific portions are epitopes. So one has a potential network of interactions available to control the reaction to antigen.

We will neglect real space dependence of populations but focus on the tag or shape variable x characterizing an antigen or epitope; call its concentration $c(x, t)$. On the other hand, we can denote the Ag-recognizing B-cell with its subsequent interaction cascade by the combining portion or *paratope* of the Ab molecule that it displays; the density of these cells will be $\rho(y, t)$. A y-cell will also expose idiotope x with accessibility $w(x, y)$, whose excision may deactivate the Ab-producing process. Hence for external antigen $a_0(x, t)$, we have

$$(6.1) \qquad c(x, t) = a_0(x, t) + \int w(x, y)\rho(y, t)dy$$

(dy is the volume in y-space, whatever its dimensionality). Now suppose antigen x binds with y on the Ig of a y-receptor at rate $B(x, y)$—thereby removing x from the system, be it true Ag or epitope—and that the binding of x produces a growth signal, allowing for time delay, of $E(y, x, t - t')$ to the growth rate of the y-population. If the rate depends on the activation signal

$$(6.2) \qquad h(y, t) = \int B(y, x)E(y, x, t - t')c(x, t')dx \, dt'$$

according to the standard multibinding curve

$$(6.3) \qquad \text{rate}_y = f_y(h(y, t)),$$

89

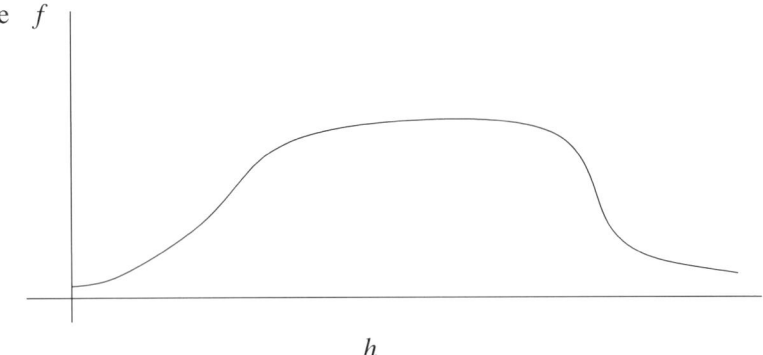

FIGURE 6.1. Model two-threshold function.

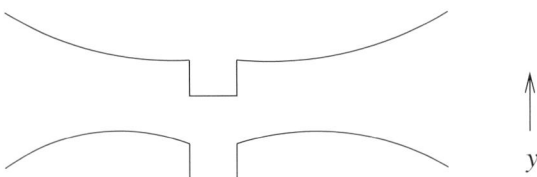

FIGURE 6.2. Complementarity detection model.

we then have its contribution to the rate equation

$$\dot{\rho}(y,t) = \cdots$$

(6.4)
$$+ \rho(y,t) f_y \left(\int B(y,x) E(y,x,t-t') \big(a_0(x,t') + w(x,z)\rho(z,t') dz \big) dx \right)$$

$$+ \cdots.$$

Introducing autonomous birth and death rates, and adopting simplifying notation, we end up with

$$\dot{\rho}(y,t) = \alpha(y,t)$$

(6.5)
$$+ \rho(y,t) \left[f_y \left(a(y,t) + \int K(y,z,t-t')\rho(z,t')dz \right) - \mu(y,t) \right].$$

To get a qualitative picture of this system, which, even in the present well-mixed (spatially uniform) approximation, is governed by an enormous number of parameters, let us carry out some sweeping simplifications: we set $\alpha(y,t) = \alpha$, $\mu(y,t) = \mu$, which we scale to 1, neglect time delay, and assume no activation externally, $a(y,t) = 0$, so that only the self-excitation of the system is in question. Thus, we write

(6.6)
$$\dot{\rho}(y) = \alpha + \rho(y) \left(f_y \left(\int K(y,z)\rho(z)dz \right) - 1 \right).$$

In fact, as an entree into the general characteristics of such a connected system, we will specialize even further: drop the y-dependence of f_y, imagine that the complementaritydetecting $K(y,z)$ can be represented by a one-dimensional cartoon

(Figure 6.2) in which only the effective amplitude of a surface feature matters,

$$(6.7) \qquad K(y, z) = g(y + z),$$

where the argument of f is scaled so that $\int g(z)dz = 1$, i.e., for uniform $\rho(y)$, $\int g(y + z)\rho\, dz = \rho$. Hence

$$(6.8) \qquad \dot{\rho}(y) = \alpha + \rho(y)\left[f\left(\int g(y + z)\rho(y)dz \right) - 1 \right].$$

To be definite, we choose f as an explicit two-threshold function (Figure 6.1)

$$(6.9) \qquad f(h) = pf_0(h), \quad f_0(h) = \frac{h}{\theta_1 + h}\frac{\theta_2}{\theta_2 + h}, \quad \theta_1 < \theta_2.$$

Now let us investigate the repertoire of (6.8). First, uniformity (at least local) in y, $\rho(y, t) = \bar{\rho}(t)$, so that in equilibrium

$$(6.10) \qquad 0 = \alpha + \bar{\rho}(pf_0(\bar{\rho}) - 1).$$

For this to be a low $\bar{\rho}$ virgin state, $\bar{\rho} \ll \theta$, or $f_0(\bar{\rho}) \sim \bar{\rho}/\theta_1$. Hence, $\bar{\rho}^2 - \bar{\rho} + \alpha = 0$, having a solution $\bar{\rho} > 0$ only if

$$(6.11) \qquad 4\alpha p < \theta_1, \quad \text{virgin state},$$

and then indeed $\bar{\rho} \sim \alpha \ll \theta_1$. Immune *proliferative* and *suppressed* states correspond to large $\bar{\rho}$, hence $pf_0(\bar{\rho}) - 1 = -\alpha/\bar{\rho} \sim 0$, or

$$(6.12) \qquad f(\bar{\rho}) = \frac{1}{p} \begin{cases} \text{proliferative} \\ \text{suppressed,} \end{cases}$$

a solution requiring that

$$(6.12') \qquad p \geq 1.$$

There are now two possibilities. For proliferation, we want $f_0(\bar{\rho} + \Delta h) > f_0(\bar{\rho})$ for $\Delta h > 0$, putting us on the rising portion $f_0(\bar{\rho}) \simeq \bar{\rho}/(\theta_1 + \bar{\rho})$, or

$$(6.13) \qquad \bar{\rho} = \frac{\theta_1}{p - 1} \quad \text{(proliferative)}$$

For suppression, it's the falling part, where $f_0(\bar{\rho}) \simeq \theta_2/\theta_2 + p$, so

$$(6.14) \qquad \bar{\rho} = (p - 1)\theta_2 \quad \text{(suppressed)}.$$

But when is the uniform state $\bar{\rho}(y) = \bar{\rho}$ stable under uniform perturbations? With $\bar{\rho}(t) = \bar{\rho} + \delta\bar{\rho}(t)$, we have from (6.8)

$$(6.15) \qquad \delta\dot{\rho} = (pf_0(\bar{\rho}) + p\bar{\rho}f_0'(\bar{\rho}) - 1)\delta\bar{\rho},$$

so that stability requires

$$(6.15') \qquad p(f_0(\bar{\rho}) + \bar{\rho}f_0'(\bar{\rho})) < 1.$$

Checking the three equilibria in order:

Virgin: low $\bar{\rho} = \alpha$, $f_0(\alpha) = \alpha/\theta_1$, $f_0'(\alpha) = 1/\theta_1$, so stability requires $2p\alpha < \theta_1$ — *always* holds.

Immune: $\bar{\rho} = \theta_1/p - 1$, $f_0(\bar{\rho}) = \bar{\rho}/(\theta_1 + \bar{\rho})$, $f_0'(\bar{\rho}) = \theta_1/(\theta_1 + \bar{\rho})^2$, requiring $(p - 1)/p < 0$ *and* $p > 1$—*never* valid.

Suppressed: $\bar{\rho} = (p-1)\theta_2$, $f_0(\bar{\rho}) = \theta_2/\theta_2 + \bar{\rho}$, $f_0'(\bar{\rho}) = -\theta_2(\theta_2 + \bar{\rho})^2$, whence $(p-1)/p < 0$ and $p > 1$—*always* stable.

More significantly, is the uniform state stable under perturbation? Without loss of generality, we take

(6.16)
$$\delta\rho(y,t) = e^{\lambda t}(\beta e^{iky} + \beta^* e^{-iky}).$$

Thus

$$\delta\dot{\rho}(y,t) = (pf_0(\bar{\rho}) - 1)\delta\rho(y,t) + p\bar{\rho}f_0'(\bar{\rho})\int g(y+z)\delta\rho(z,t)dz$$

$$= (pf_0(\bar{\rho}) - 1)\delta\rho(y,t) + \bar{\rho}pf_0'(\bar{\rho})(\beta e^{-iky} + \beta^* e^{iky})\tilde{g}(k)e^{\lambda t}$$

where $\tilde{g}(k) = \int e^{iky}g(z)dz$, which is assumed real (e.g., $\tilde{g}(k) = e^{-(1/2)\sigma^2 k^2}$ for a Gaussian g). Equating coefficients of e^{iky} and e^{-iky},

(6.17)
$$\beta(pf_0(\bar{\rho}) - 1 - \lambda) + \beta^* p\bar{\rho}f_0'(\bar{\rho})\tilde{g}(k) = 0,$$
$$\beta^*(pf_0(\bar{\rho}) - 1 - \lambda) + \beta p\bar{\rho}f_0'(\bar{\rho})\tilde{g}(k) = 0.$$

Conjugating the second equation and comparing, $\beta(\lambda^* - \lambda) = 0$, so λ is real. Further, setting $\beta = \beta_0 + i\beta_1$,

(6.18)
$$\beta_0(pf_0(\bar{\rho}) - 1 - \lambda + p\bar{\rho}f_0'(\bar{\rho})\tilde{g}(k)) = 0,$$
$$\beta_1(pf_0(\bar{\rho}) - 1 - \lambda - p\bar{\rho}f_0'(\bar{\rho})\tilde{g}(k)) = 0,$$

leading to the two possibilities

(6.19)
$$\beta_0 = 0, \ \lambda = \lambda^- \quad \text{or} \quad \beta_1 = 0, \ \lambda = \lambda^+$$
$$\text{where } \lambda^{\pm} = pf_0(\bar{\rho}) - 1 \pm p\bar{\rho}f_0'(\bar{\rho})\tilde{g}(k).$$

Stability requires $\lambda < 0$ for both $\lambda^{\pm}$, and so we have:

Virgin: $\bar{\rho} \sim \alpha$, $f_0(\bar{\rho}) \sim \bar{\rho}/\theta_1$, $\lambda^{\pm} = \frac{\alpha p}{\theta_1} - 1 \pm \frac{\alpha p}{\theta_1}\tilde{g}(k)$. Now $\tilde{g}(0) = 1 > \tilde{g}(k \neq 0)$ and $\alpha p < \frac{\theta_1}{4}$, so it is unstable only for $\lambda^+ > 0$, with $k = 0$ as the worst case. But $\lambda^+(0) = \frac{2\alpha p}{\theta_1} - 1 < 0$, so it is *stable* against nonuniform perturbations as well.

Immune: $\bar{\rho} = \frac{\theta_1}{p-1}$; we can let $\alpha \to 0$, so $f_0(\bar{\rho}) = \frac{1}{p}$, $f_0'(\bar{\rho}) = \frac{(p-1)^2}{\theta_1 p^2}$ and $\lambda^{\pm} = \pm\frac{p-1}{p}\tilde{g}(k)$, which is *unstable* at all k to λ^+, i.e., $\delta\rho\alpha e^{\lambda^+ t}\cos ky$ as an extension of the $k = 0$ self-stimulation.

Suppressed: $\bar{\rho} = (p-1)\theta_2$, $\alpha \to 0$, $f_0(\bar{\rho}) = \frac{1}{p}$, $f_0'(\bar{\rho}) = -\frac{1}{p^2}\theta_2$, and $\lambda^{\pm} = \mp\frac{p-1}{p}\tilde{g}(k)$, which is *unstable* at all k to $\lambda^- = \delta\rho \sim e^{\lambda^- t}\sin ky$.

In order for the exponential population instability to saturate, one needs a weak logistic term, e.g.,

(6.20)
$$\dot{\rho} = \alpha + \rho(pf_0(k)r(\rho) - 1) \quad \text{where } r(\rho) = \frac{\theta_3}{\theta_3 + \rho},$$

and indeed numerical solution shows that one then ends up with clusters larger than the range of $g(z)$, either immune or suppressed, in a sea of virgin components. The crucial driving force here is, of course, the binding strength $g(y+z)$

with its one-dimensional characterization of cell type. Generalization to high-dimensional continuous species space and to discrete subspaces of biomolecular strings (e.g., Cayley tree lattice) with realistic complementation have been carried out as well, resulting in a huge class of dynamic behaviors. Clearly, more specific sets of molecular signatures—those evolutionarily developed—should be used.

6.2. Estimates of Connectivity

The mutually activated but tolerant state that has been suggested is a mechanism for keeping the immune system under control. In fact, it has been estimated that some 10–30% of the immune system consists of self-recognizing subpopulations. The normal ones tend to express the pentamer IgM, whereas autoimmune malfunction tends to emphasize IgG (monomer or dimer). A conceptual division has been made distinguishing *allopoetic*, which reacts to external Ag, so clonal deletion is crucial, and *autopoetic*, for which internal reactions remain that cause pathology.

As a minimal model for the B-network, let b_i designate the concentration of cell-bound Ab of type i, a_i as the corresponding free Ab. By assuming a symmetric bilinear binding function with affinity matrix J_{ij}, the activation

$$(6.21) \qquad h_i = \sum_j J_{ij} b_j$$

then gives rise (with suitable scaling) to

$$(6.22) \qquad \begin{aligned} \dot{a}_i &= -a_i + M(h_i) b_i, \\ \dot{b}_i &= -b_i + P(h_i) b_i, \end{aligned}$$

where M and P are maturation and proliferation functions whose precise form is not crucial. The matrix J_{ij} was determined empirically for a sample of 26 clones in a mouse, divided into a distribution of small and large affinities. Two numerical dynamical studies were run, the first unstimulated, i.e., using (6.21) and (6.22). The result was that one could divide the clone types into four classes: A, multiaffinity; B and C, moderate affinity; D, weak affinity. One then finds that for A, there were small cycles in the (a_i, b_i) phase flow; for B and C, clear limit cycles; for D, silent (stationary) asymptotics. In the second numerical study, species k was stimulated externally at amplitude α:

$$(6.23) \qquad h_i = \sum J_{ij} a_j + \alpha \delta_{ik}.$$

This resulted in
So high connectivity resulted in high tolerance.

6.3. Cytokine Networks

It is not clear that extensive cell-cell networks are the norm for immune system operation. But a dense network of communication and consequent gene activation via cytokines, or intercellular messengers, appears to be universal for all cell types. A given cytokine can bind to a number of different receptor types, and receptors,

$k \in D$:   poorly connected clones exploded, others not affected

$k \in B$ or C: moderately connected part:
                    activation integrated into cyclic behavior,
                    but eventual explosion

$k \in B$ or C: well connected part:
                    activity under control, but spreads to whole network

$k \in A$:   virtually no change in behavior.

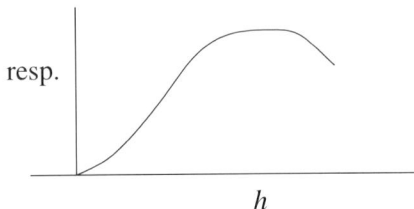

FIGURE 6.3. Typical response function.

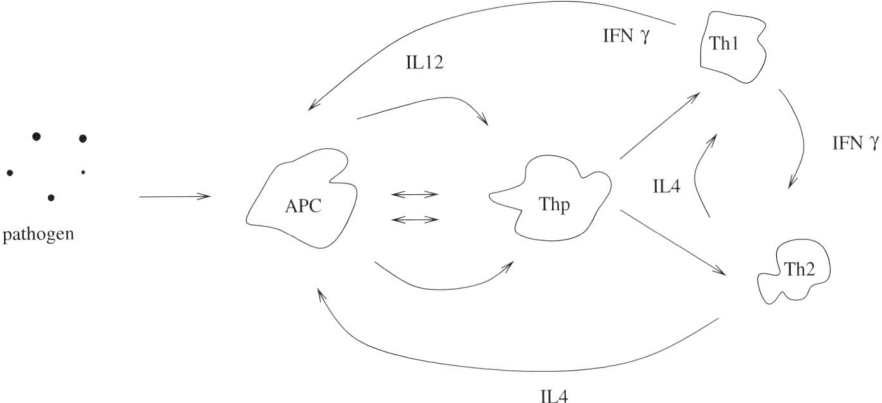

FIGURE 6.4. Cartoon of network.

often with a modular sturcture, can bind different cytokines as well. The response appears in general to follow the now-familiar two-threshold form (Figure 6.3), but not dramatically.

One of the most studied components of the cytokine regulatory system is that involved in T-cell precursor differentiation to Th1 and Th2 subclasses. This is about as simple a network as one could imagine, insofar as it is reducible to the study of two components, but it is enough to introduce some of the principal phenomenology. Th1 cells are responsible for cell-mediated immune response and inflammation, Th2 for Ab production, including allergic reactions. They are both differentiated from precursor T-cells (Thp), and clearly the wrong response to a signal can be devastating. Now their maturation is determined by the cytokines they (as well as APCs) themselves secrete, so one has very much of a network.

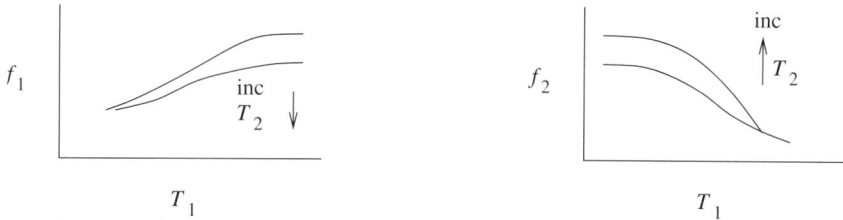

FIGURE 6.5. Activation level dependence. T_1 and T_2 denote the Th1 and Th2 concentrations.

In broad summary, by inserting local (Michaelis-Menten) equilibrium for the concentrations of the Th1 and Th2 "compartments," the corresponding cytokine flow (Figure 6.4) then can be modeled as obeying the chemical kinetics

$$\dot{T}_1 = a_1 + f_1(T_1, T_2) - \mu_1 T_1,$$
$$\dot{T}_2 = a_2 + f_2(T_1, T_2) - \mu_2 T_2,$$

(6.24)

where f_1 would be stimulated by T_1, inhibited by T_2, and conversely for f_2. The activation signals a_1 and a_2, and death rates μ_1 and μ_2, would in fact be T_1- and T_2-dependent as well. A model form that has been used (Figure 6.5) is

$$f_1(T_1, T_2) = \frac{\beta_1 T_1}{1 + \alpha_2 T_2},$$
$$f_2(T_1, T_2) = \frac{\beta_2 T_2}{1 + \alpha_1 T_1 + \alpha_2 T_2}.$$

(6.25)

The analysis of the repertoire as a function of the activation levels is straightforward but involved. In general, one proceeds by plotting the *nullclines* $\dot{T}_1 = 0$ and $\dot{T}_2 = 0$; these point to the equilibrium states and compartmentalize the phase plane, allowing a rapid description of trajectories (Figure 6.6).

For example, with no activation by Ag, one has a single stable equilibrium point that attracts trajectories. With T_1 activation alone, the behavior is as shown, a separatrix now appearing through the new saddle point. And with activation along both channels, three saddle points make for a still more complex repertoire, suggesting however, how one might try to control Th1/Th2 incited pathologies, inflammation, allergy, etc.

References for Chapter 6

Bergmann, C., van Hemmen, J. L., and Segel, L. A. Th1 or Th2: how an appropriate T helper response can be made. *Bull. Math. Bio.* 63(3): 405–430, 2001. doi:10.1006/bulm.2000.0215

Callard, R., George, A. J. T., and Stark, J. Cytokines, chaos, and complexity. *Immunity* 11(5): 507–513, 1999. doi:10.1016/S1074-7613(00)80125-9

de Boer, R. J., Segel, L. A., and Perelson, A. S. Pattern formation in one- and two-dimensional shape-space models of the immune system. *J. Theor. Bio.* 155(3): 295–333, 1992.

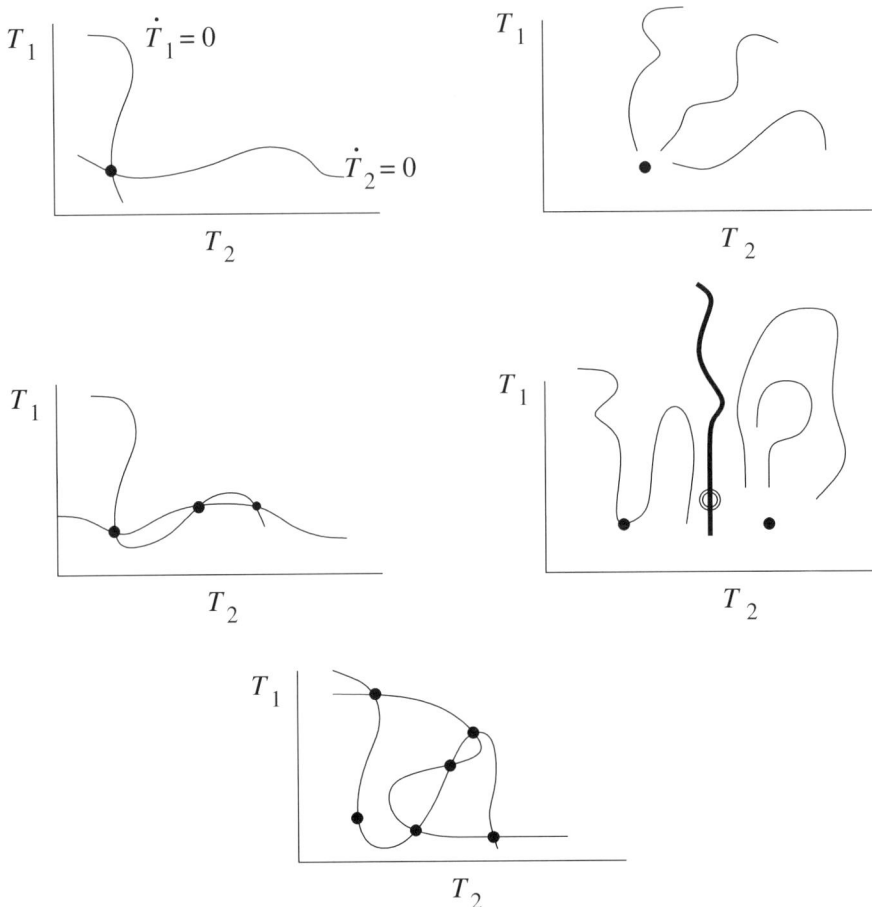

FIGURE 6.6. Activation trajectories.

Stewart, J., Varela, F. J., and Coutinho, A. The relationship between connectivity and tolerance as revealed by computer simulation of the immune network: Some lessons for an understanding of autoimmunity. *J. Autoimmunity* 2: supp. 1, 15–23, 1989. doi:10.1016/0896-8411(89)90113-3

CHAPTER 7

Viewpoint of the Virus

7.1. Reprise

When only one molecule is involved, reproduction can be a fairly simple process. When the organism is a highly correlated set of molecules, this is no longer the case, and much more elaborate machinery is required. Viruses are consummate parasites: they cheat and use another organism's machinery for this purpose, so they can travel light. Of course, little fleas have smaller fleas; viroids—RNA only some 3×10^2 nucleotides long—hitch a ride on viruses to take advantage of the latter's usurping a cell's reproduction machinery.

Viruses are incapable of replication, transcription, or translation outside of a host cell. Structurally, virions above the viroid level go from 20–300 nm in size, 1–300 kb in nucleotide content on their genomes, typically have a protein coat or capsid, may or may not have a lipoprotein envelope, and may or may not have protein in place to aid the cell's transcription and replication of their genomes. The genomic material can be RNA or DNA, double strand or single strand, or two copies (diploid) of a single strand in the RNA case; the single RNA strand can have positive sense (as in the host's mRNA), negative, or ambi (both). The shape is that of the outer skin, capsid, or envelope: icosahedral as in poliovirus (generally having some multiple of 60 units); enveloped icosahedral as in herpes; complex with tail as in phage T4 (see Figure 7.1); helical, as in phage MK3 or TMV; or enveloped helical, as in rhabdovirus.

As to general strategy, small DNA viruses use both the cell's genome and its molecular servants to replicate; larger ones often encode their own polymerases. RNA viruses *must* encode their own RNA-dependent polymerases (the host cell won't have them) or, as in retroviruses, RNA-dependent polymerases are encoded

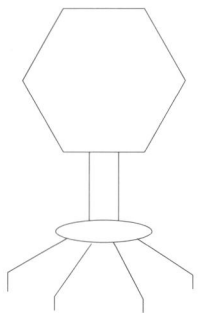

FIGURE 7.1. T4 cartoon.

(reverse transcriptase) to replicate via the host DNA. Enveloped virions get their
envelopes: icosahedral as in poliovirus (generally having some multiple of 60
units); envelope by budding from the host membrane; they generally have glyco-
protein "antireceptors" to bind to receptors on the host. In general, the one-strand
genome can be linear, circular, or segmented (looking like a double strand); when
segmented, or actually diploid, one can have rearrangement inside the virion, as
in familiar chromosomal crossing over, giving rise to fast evolution. Even if not,
they—especially lentiviruses such as HIV—have frequent mutations, i.e., mistakes
in replication, allowing them to meet environmental changes but also keeping them
from getting so large as to make lethal errors too often.

Viruses just try to multiply, but in the process they may be virulent—kill the
host cell—by competing for enzymes and growth factors, damaging cell mem-
branes, etc., at too fast a rate. Thus, evolutionary development of controls over
their rate of replication is mandatory to maximize total reproduction rate.

7.2. Short-Time Strategy

We have seen that the immune system and the pathogen are in an evolutionary
battle that is closely matched. Let us close by returning to the HIV virus, initiator
of so much immunological research. We confine our discussion to two topics that
are of course not restricted to HIV.

HIV is very much on the attack against the crucial CD4$^+$ T-cells of the mammalian immune system. When it infects a cell, the host obligingly produces hun-
dreds to thousands of new virions before it succumbs to membrane depletion, viral
protein buildup, and the like. It is certainly in the short-term interest of the virus to
adjust its replication rate to maximize the burst size—the total virions produced—
before the cell dies, and in particular it had better not kill the cell too fast (at longer
time, it will be the number of virions produced per unit time in the host population
that matters). To see the nature of the optimum replication schedule that would
come about during viral evolution, we have to model the mortality rate of a cell.
Suppose

$$I(t) = \text{size of infected population at time } t \text{ (after infection)},$$
$$N(t) = \text{number of virions produced until } t,$$
$$P = \text{production rate, virions/cell/unit time},$$
$$\mu = \text{cell mortality rate/unit time}.$$

A particularly simple model proceeds by imagining that N itself is a good
measure of physiological time, since it both measures accumulated damage and
the increasing virally induced protein complement of the cell, which could well
serve as a quantitative signal. In this case, we would have a given $\mu(N, P)$ and
would seek the viral strategy $P(N)$.

Our system is then simply (normalized to one initial cell)

$$(7.1) \qquad \dot{N} = PI, \quad \dot{I} = -\mu I, \quad I(0) = 1,$$

which we write as

$$
(7.2) \qquad \frac{dI}{dN} = -\frac{\mu(N, P(N))}{P(N)}
$$

and integrate to obtain

$$
(7.3) \qquad I(N) = 1 - \int_0^N \frac{\mu(N, P(N'))}{P(N')}\, dN'.
$$

The burst size $\bar{N}$ is the value of N where $I = 0$, and so $\bar{N}$ is determined by

$$
(7.4) \qquad \int_0^{\bar{N}} \frac{\mu(N, P(N))}{P(N)}\, dN = 1.
$$

To maximize $\bar{N}$, given the fixed form of the integral, we of course want to select $P(N)$ to minimize the integrand at each value of N:

$$
(7.5) \qquad \begin{aligned}
\frac{\partial}{\partial P(N)} \frac{\mu(N, P(N))}{P(N)} &= 0, \\
\frac{\partial^2}{\partial P(N)^2} \frac{\mu(N, P(N))}{P(N)} &\geq 0.
\end{aligned}
$$

For example, if $\mu(N, P) = \mu(N) + \gamma^2 P^2$, a sum of intrinsic and induced mortality rates, this yields

$$
(7.6) \qquad P(N) = \frac{1}{\gamma} \mu(N)^{1/2},
$$

and from (7.4)

$$
(7.7) \qquad \int_0^{\bar{N}} \mu(N)^{1/2}\, dN = \frac{1}{2\gamma}
$$

determines $\bar{N}$—just $1/(2\gamma\mu^{1/2})$ for constant μ. The actual time dependence can now be recovered as well: in the special case of $\mu(N) = \mu$, $I(N) = 1 - 2\gamma\mu^{1/2}N$, so $dt = -\frac{1}{\mu} dI/I$, $I = e^{-2\mu t}$, and $N = (1 - e^{-2\mu t})/2\gamma\mu^{1/2}$.

The above model is far from unique. Another possibility is to imagine that μ in fact depends upon physical time as $\mu(t, P)$ and seek the maximizing $P(t)$. Here the probability of a cell surviving until t is

$$
(7.8) \qquad \sigma(t) = e^{-\int_0^t \mu(\tau, P(\tau)) d\tau},
$$

and the burst size is simply

$$
(7.9) \qquad N[P] = \int_0^\infty P(t) e^{-\int_0^t \mu(\tau, P(\tau)) d\tau}\, dt.
$$

The functional $N(P)$ is to be maximized by choice of $\{P(t)\}$, presumably subject to a biological restriction $P(t) \leq P_M$.

EXAMPLE 1. $\mu(P) = \lambda P$, so $N[P] = \frac{1}{\lambda}(1 - \epsilon^{-\lambda \int_0^\infty P(t)\,dt})$, and all nonintegrable $\{P(t)\}$ give the same maximum $N[P] = \frac{1}{\lambda}$.

EXAMPLE 2. $\mu[P] = m + \lambda P$, now including an intrinsic mortality rate, so that (show this!)

$$N[P] = \frac{1}{\lambda}\left(1 - m \int_0^\infty e^{-mt}\, e^{-\lambda \int_0^t P(\tau)\,d\tau}\, dt\right),$$

and we must have $P = P_M$ at all times, giving $N[P] = P_M/(m + \lambda P_M)$, which agrees with Example 1 when $m \to 0$.

EXAMPLE 3. Maximum $N[P]$ is stationary under changes in the function $P(t)$; suppose we ignore the P_M restriction in checking this. Then from (7.9) we have

$$\delta N[P] = \int_0^\infty \delta P(t)e^{-\int_0^t \mu(\tau',p(\tau))d\tau'}\, dt$$
$$- \int_0^\infty P(t)\int_0^t \mu'_P(\tau, P(\tau))\delta P(\tau)d\tau\, e^{-\int_0^t \mu(\tau',P(\tau'))d\tau'}\, dt.$$

Here $0 \le \tau \le t < \infty$, so interchanging t and τ in the second integral, we have

(7.10)
$$\delta N(P) = \int_0^\infty \delta P(t)\left[e^{-\int_0^t \mu(\tau',P(\tau'))d\tau'} \right.$$
$$\left. - \int_t^\infty P(t)\mu'_P(t, P(t))e^{-\int_0^\tau \mu(\tau',P(\tau'))d\tau'}\right]dt.$$

Thus, max $N[P]$ requires $\delta N(P) = 0$, or

$$e^{-\int_0^t \mu(\tau',P(\tau'))d\tau'} = \mu'_P(t, P(t)) \int_t^\infty P(t)e^{-\int_0^t \mu(\tau',P(\tau'))d\tau'}d\tau;$$

taking $\partial/\partial t$ and canceling the exponential, we obtain

$$-\frac{\mu(t, P(t))}{\mu'_P(t, P(t))} - \frac{\partial}{\partial t}\frac{\mu'_P(t, P(t))}{\mu'_P(t, P(t))^2} = -P(t),$$

which we write as

(7.11)
$$\frac{dP}{dt} = \frac{1}{\mu''_{PP}(t, P(t))}$$
$$\times \left[\mu'_P(t, P(t))^2\left(P(t) - \frac{\mu(t, P(t))}{\mu'_P(t, P(t))}\right) - \frac{\partial^2\mu(t, P(t))}{\partial P\, \partial t}\right].$$

The prototypical special case is now $\mu(t, P) = m(t) + \frac{\lambda}{2}P^2$. We can easily integrate (7.11), here reducing to $\dot{P} = \frac{\lambda}{2}P^3 - mP$, and find

(7.12)
$$P(t) = e^{-\int_0^t m(\tau)dt}\left(\frac{1}{P(0)^2} - \int_0^t e^{-3\int_0^\tau m(\tau')d\tau'}\, d\tau\right)^{-1/2}.$$

Interestingly, this depends sensitively on $P(0)$ and in fact blows up at finite time if

(7.13)
$$P(0) > \left(\int_0^\infty e^{-3\int_0^\tau m(\tau')d\tau'}\, d\tau\right)^{-1/2},$$

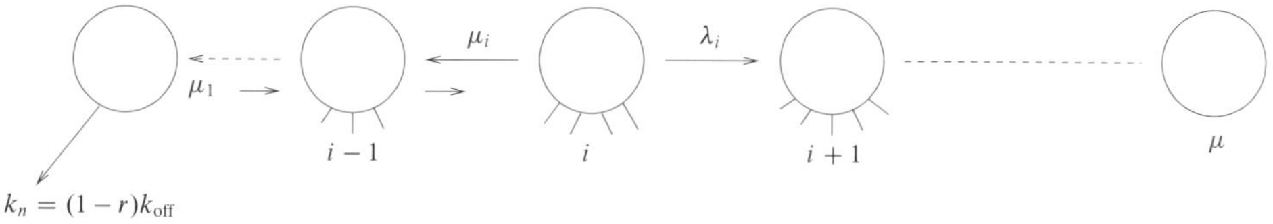

FIGURE 7.2. Model of APC antigen retention.

meaning of course that the neglected P_M has taken over. So there is a nontrivial phenomenology.

Homework Assignment 12

(1) What happens in the (7.4) analysis when $(\partial^2/\partial P^2)\mu(N, P)/P \geq 0$ is not always true?

7.3. Intermediate Time Control

Various HIV treatments stop the production of virus but do not eliminate virus being held internally in cells. T4 cells die, so it doesn't matter. But follicular dendritic cells (FDCs) in lymphoid tissue are antigen-presenting cells (APCs) whose job it is to hold onto small amounts of antigen to serve as signal when needed, and this is held on the surface, so the cell doesn't die. Gradually the viral antigen detaches (it actually represents immune system complement deposited on the virus, and this binds to complement receptors on the APC), but meanwhile it can serve as a new source of virus when a T-cell meets an FDC, and so can be a large intermediate-time reservoir. How important is this?

In the model we will use (Figure 7.2), a virion has n sites it can use for attachment to any of the very large number R_T of mobile receptor sites on the FDC.

$$
\begin{aligned}
\lambda_i &= (n - i)k_+ R_T, \\
\mu_i &= i k_- \quad \text{for } 2 \leq i \leq \cdots \leq n, \\
\mu_1 &= k_r = (1 - \gamma)k_{\text{off}}, \\
k_{\text{off}} &= \text{last bond's } k_-, \\
\gamma &= \text{probability of last bond rebinding before diffusing away.}
\end{aligned}
$$
(7.14)

We now examine the $\{t_i\}$, the mean waiting times for a virion to "escape" when i of its n sites are initially bound. These can be found indirectly by looking at the first-passage time to unbinding in the chemical kinetics with initial i sites bound, or equivalently and directly, from the obvious

$$
\begin{aligned}
t_0 &= 0, \\
t_i &= \frac{1}{\lambda_i + \mu_i} + \left(\frac{\lambda_i}{\lambda_i + \mu_i}\right)t_{i+1} + \left(\frac{\mu_i}{\lambda_i + \mu_i}\right)t_{i-1} \quad \text{for } i = 1, \ldots, n - 1, \\
t_n &= \frac{1}{\mu_n} + t_{n-1}
\end{aligned}
$$
(7.15)

(when the state disappears from i, at rate $\lambda_i + \mu_i$, it either appears at $i + 1$, with probability $\lambda_i / (\lambda_i + \mu_i)$, or at $i - 1$, with probability $\mu_i / (\lambda_i + \mu_i)$, and picks up the associated waiting time). The recursion relation (7.15) can be written as $\mu_i (t_i - t_{i-1}) = 1 + \lambda_i (t_{i+1} - t_i)$, or simply that

$$(7.16) \qquad t_i - t_{i-1} = \frac{1}{\mu_i} + \frac{\lambda_i}{\mu_i}(t_{i+1} - t_i).$$

In particular, we have

$$
\begin{aligned}
t_1 &= \frac{1}{\mu_1} + \frac{\lambda_1}{\mu_1}(t_2 - t_1) \\
&= \frac{1}{\mu_1} + \frac{\lambda_1}{\mu_1}\left(\frac{1}{\mu_2} + \frac{\lambda_2}{\mu_2}(t_3 - t_2)\right) \\
(7.17) \quad &= \frac{1}{\mu_1} + \frac{\lambda_1}{\mu_1}\left(\frac{1}{\mu_2} + \frac{\lambda_2}{\mu_2}\left(\frac{1}{\mu_3} + \frac{\lambda_3}{\mu_3}(t_4 - t_3)\right)\right) \\
&\;\;\vdots \\
&= \frac{1}{\mu_1} + \frac{\lambda_1}{\mu_1 \mu_2} + \frac{\lambda_1 \lambda_2}{\mu_1 \mu_2 \mu_3} + \cdots + \frac{\lambda_1 \lambda_2}{\mu_1 \mu_2}\cdots\frac{\lambda_{n-1}}{\mu_{n-1}}(t_n - t_{n-1}),
\end{aligned}
$$

or

$$
\begin{aligned}
(7.18) \qquad t_1 &= \frac{1}{\mu_1}\left(1 + \sum_{k=1}^{n-1} \frac{(n-1)\ldots(n-k)}{(k+1)!}\left(\frac{k_+}{k_-}R_T\right)^k\right) \\
&= \frac{1}{k_1}\frac{(1+\alpha)^n - 1}{n\alpha} \quad \text{where } \alpha = \frac{k_+}{k_-}R_T.
\end{aligned}
$$

Similarly, for $i > 1$, we find

$$(7.19) \qquad t_i = t_1 + \frac{1}{k_1}\left[\sum_{j=2}^{i}\frac{1}{j} + \sum_{j=2}^{i}\sum_{k=1}^{n-j}\frac{(n-j)!/(n-j-k)!}{(j+k)!/(j-1)!}\alpha^k\right].$$

For the worst-case scenario, we of course have to look at

$$(7.20) \qquad t_n = t_1 \sum_{j=1}^{n}\sum_{k=0}^{n-j}\frac{(n-j)!(j-1)!}{(n-j-k)!(j+k)!}\alpha^k.$$

We will see that, amazingly, $t_n \sim t_1$. Here's how (not the simplest way but illustrating valuable techniques): In a sum, it's always nice to have binomial coefficients, so let's rewrite (7.20) as

$$(7.21) \qquad t_n = \frac{1}{k_1}\sum_{j=1}^{n}\sum_{k=0}^{n-j}\binom{n-j}{k}\frac{k!(j-1)!}{(j+k)!}\alpha^k.$$

But then we recognize the beta function

$$(7.22) \qquad \frac{k(j-1)!}{(j+k)!} = \frac{\Gamma(k+1)\Gamma(j)}{\Gamma(j+k+1)} = \int_0^1 x^k(1-x)^{j-1}\,dx,$$

allowing us to rewrite

$$t_n = \frac{1}{k_1} \int_0^1 \sum_{j=1}^n \sum_{k=0}^{n-j} \binom{n-j}{k} x^k (1-x)^{j-1} \alpha^k \, dx$$

$$= \frac{1}{k_1} \int_0^1 \sum_{j=1}^n (1-x)^{j-1} (1-\alpha x)^{n-j} \, dx$$

$$(7.23) \qquad = \frac{1}{k_1} \int_0^1 ((1+\alpha x)^n - (1-x)^n) dx / x(\alpha+1).$$

The parameter $1 + \alpha$ is more convenient, and so we further transform

$$t_n = \frac{1}{k_1} \int_0^1 \frac{(x(\alpha+1)+1-x)^n - (1-x)^n}{x(\alpha+x)} \, dx$$

$$(7.24) \qquad = \frac{1}{k_1} \int \sum_{k=1}^n \binom{n}{k} x^{k-1} (1+\alpha)^{k-1} (1-x)^{n-k} \, dx$$

$$= \frac{1}{k_1} \sum_{k=1}^n \frac{(1+\alpha)^{k-1}}{k} = \frac{1}{k_1} \sum_{j=0}^{n-1} \frac{(1+\alpha)^{n-1-j}}{n-k},$$

which is pretty neat. Now we can get to work.

Of course, we are interested in large n, and it would be nice to get an upper bound as an expansion in $1/n$. A not very good one is gotten from

$$(7.25) \qquad \frac{1}{n-j} \le \frac{j+1}{n}$$

(for $i < n$), which can be checked at once. But this can also be used in an iteration, starting with

$$(7.26) \qquad \frac{1}{n-j} = \frac{1}{n} + \frac{j}{n} \frac{1}{n-j}$$

$$\le \frac{1}{n} + \frac{j(j+1)}{n^2},$$

which will be good enough.

Plugging (7.26) into (7.24), we get

$$(7.27) \qquad t_n \le \frac{1}{k_1} \sum_{j=0}^{n-1} \frac{(1+\alpha)^{n-1-j}}{n} + \frac{1}{k_1} \sum_{j=0}^{n-1} \frac{1}{n^2} j(j+1)(1+\alpha)^{n-1-j}.$$

For the first part,

$$\frac{1}{k_1} \sum_{j=0}^{n-1} \frac{(1+\alpha)^{n-1-j}}{n} = \frac{1}{k_1} \frac{(1+\alpha)^n - 1}{\alpha n} = t_1,$$

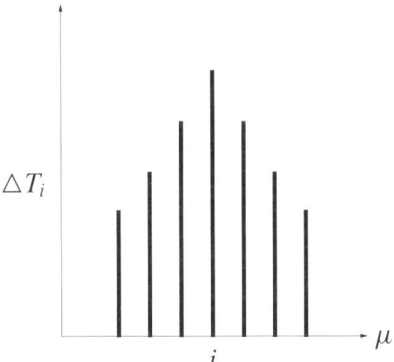

FIGURE 7.3. Site occupation.

while for the second

$$\sum_{j=0}^{n-1}(j+1)(1+\alpha)^{-(j+2)} = \frac{\partial^2}{\partial\alpha^2}\sum_{j=0}^{n-1}(1+\alpha)^{-j}.$$

Hence (7.20) tells us that

(7.28) $$t_n \le t_1 + \frac{2(1+\alpha)^{n-1}}{k_1 n^2 \alpha^3}.$$

We conclude that

(7.29) $$\frac{t_n}{t_1} \le 1 + \frac{2(1+\alpha)}{n\alpha^2[1-(1+\alpha)^{-n}]} = 1 + O(1/n) \quad \text{as } u \to \infty.$$

$$\lambda_i = (n-i)k_+ R_T,$$
$$\mu_i = i k_- \quad \text{for } 2 \le i \le \cdots \le n,$$
(7.30) $$\mu_1 = k_r = (1-\gamma)k_{\text{off}},$$
$$k_{\text{off}} = \text{last bond's } k_-,$$

$$\gamma = \text{probability of last bond rebinding before diffusing away.}$$

The reason is simple: if one looks at the distribution of times ΔT_i spent in state i (Figure 7.3) even when only one state is initially occupied, it's already concentrated about $n/2$. Sticking in parameters, FDCs can hang on to HIV for years, but B-cells—which are also APCs—lose it fast.

References for Chapter 7

Coombs, D., Gilchrist, M. A., Percus, J., and Perelson, A. S. Optimal viral production. *Bull. Math. Bio.* 65(6): 1003–1023, 2003. doi:10.1016/S0092-8240(03)00056-9

Hlavacek, W. S., Percus, J. K., Percus, O. E., Perelson, A. S., and Wofsy, C. Retention of antigen on follicular dendritic cells and B lymphocytes through complement-mediated multivalent ligand-receptor interactions: theory and application to HIV treatment. *Math Biosci.* 176(2): 185–202, 2002.

Sasaki, A., and Iwasa, Y. Optimal growth schedule of pathogens within a host: switching between lytic and latent cycles. *Theor. Popul. Bio.* 39(2): 201–239, 1991.

General References

Alberts, B., Bray, D., Lewis, J., Raff, M., Roberts, K., and Watson, J. D. *Molecular biology of the cell.* Garland, New York, 1989.

Janeway, C., Travers, P., Walport, M., and Shlomchik, M. *Immunobiology: the immune system in health and disease.* Garland, New York, 1996.

Marchuk, G. I. *Mathematical models in immunology.* Springer, Berlin, 1983.

Nowak, M. A., and May, R. *Virus dynamics: mathematical principles of immunology and virology.* Oxford, New York, 2000.

Percus, J. *Lectures on mathematics of immunology.* Courant Institute, New York University, New York, 1986.

Perelson, A. S., ed. *Theoretical immunology: The proceedings of the Theoretical Immunology Workshop, held June 1987, in Santa Fe, New Mexico.* Addison-Wesley, Redwood City, Calif., 1988.

Perelson, A. S., and Weisbuch, G. Immunology for physicists. *Rev. Mod. Phys.* 69(4): 1219–1268, 1997. doi:10.1103/RevModPhys.69.1219

Segel, L. A., and Cohen, I. R., eds. *Design principles for the immune system and distributed autonomous systems.* Sante Fe Institute Studies in the Sciences of Complexity. Oxford, New York, 2001.

Index

Titles in This Series